*Here's to the millions of unsung heroes—the men and women who work hard to put bread on the table, pay the bills, clothe their families, and hope today is a little better than yesterday. Their lives are not easy; they have to earn everything they have. Aside from their daily struggles, they show a remarkable capacity to care about life, their families, their communities, and their work. They dream of making this world a better place to live and a better place to make a living through their brains, sweat, and talents. These people are the true superstars! This book is dedicated to the past generation of working men and women who made America a great country in which to live and work. It is also dedicated to today's workers who strive to build on that greatness.*

# Contents

# Preface

Yqou and I are one among many,
but still we are one.
We cannot do everything,
but still we can do *something*.

That's what this book is about: doing *something* to enhance the quality of life for millions of people who spend one fourth of their lives at work. Worksite health promotion (WHP) is a viable, cost-effective way to combat many of the ailments and stressors that are to blame for poor health and lost productivity at the workplace. More and more companies are expected to implement the programs and strategies described in this text.

This book is written primarily for students planning careers in the field of WHP and for those who currently plan, implement, and direct WHP programs for their companies.

## HOW THIS BOOK IS ORGANIZED

No single formula exists for planning successful health promotion programs. A program for a large company with multisite operations may look very different from a program at a small company. However, common denominators do exist among successful programs. These common denominators can be affiliated with the following cornerstones: needs assessment and evaluation, healthy culture development, effective interventions, and relapse prevention.

Experts in the field have developed a framework to help program planners recognize employee needs and interests before planning and implementing appropriate WHP programs. The framework consists of five distinct, yet interrelated phases (see figure 1):

1. **Identification:** identifying health-related problems
2. **Assessment:** assessing employees' interests
3. **Planning:** locating and applying necessary resources to establish a program
4. **Implementation:** positioning, promoting, and implementing a program
5. **Evaluation:** measuring the impact of a program

Based upon the framework presented in figure 1, this book is divided into three parts, each dealing with an important area of WHP. Part I, Initiating Worksite Health Promotion, presents an overview of the economic forces affecting worksites and how employers are responding to changing demographics, employees' health risks, rising health care costs, and health-related productivity challenges. Chapter 1 defines and explains WHP and its long and rich history. Arguments for and against the concept of WHP are scrutinized. Chapter 2 covers the identification and assessment phases of the planning process.

Part II, Planning Worksite Health Promotion Programs, contains three chapters focused on front-end programming decisions. Chapter 3 explains how to plan WHP programs, including setting appropriate goals, dealing with funding and budgeting concerns, and proposing WHP plans to management. Chapter 4 describes factors to consider in selecting healthy lifestyle programs. Chapter 5 describes various options for allocating resources and provides budgetary considerations.

Part III, Accomplishing and Evaluating Worksite Health Promotion, contains three chapters that focus on employee risk-reduction strategies, program promotion, and program evaluation.

Chapter 6 describes key strategies for reducing major health risks among employees. The chapter focuses on ways in which to transform an unhealthy workplace into a health-minded culture that can promote employee health and productivity. Chapter 7, on promoting and launching WHP programs, discusses marketing issues and suggests ways to promote the programs so that they catch on and become popular with the general workforce. Chapter 8 describes the essentials of program evaluation and how to build evaluation protocols into the program itself.

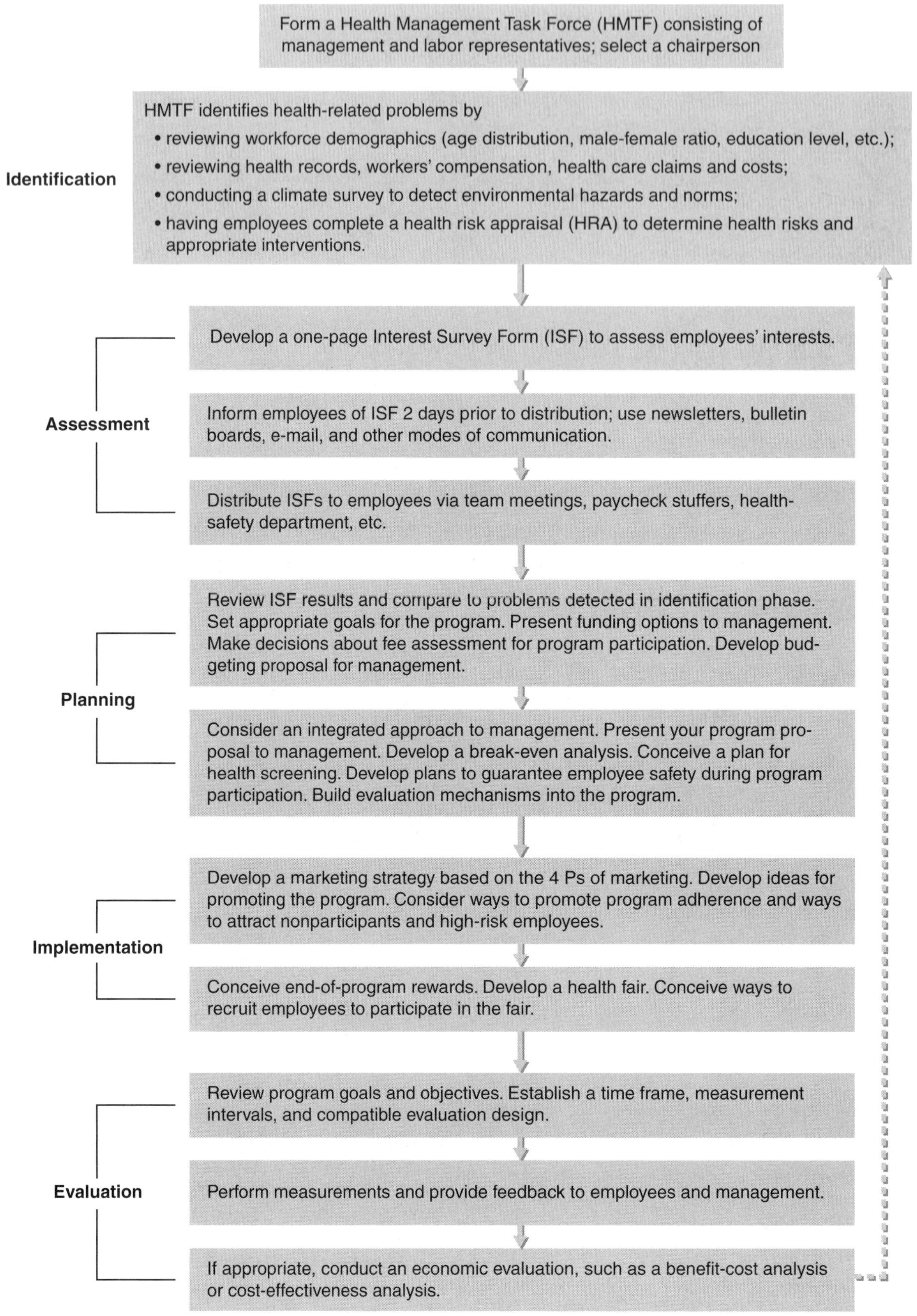

**Identification**

Form a Health Management Task Force (HMTF) consisting of management and labor representatives; select a chairperson

HMTF identifies health-related problems by
- reviewing workforce demographics (age distribution, male-female ratio, education level, etc.);
- reviewing health records, workers' compensation, health care claims and costs;
- conducting a climate survey to detect environmental hazards and norms;
- having employees complete a health risk appraisal (HRA) to determine health risks and appropriate interventions.

**Assessment**

Develop a one-page Interest Survey Form (ISF) to assess employees' interests.

Inform employees of ISF 2 days prior to distribution; use newsletters, bulletin boards, e-mail, and other modes of communication.

Distribute ISFs to employees via team meetings, paycheck stuffers, health-safety department, etc.

**Planning**

Review ISF results and compare to problems detected in identification phase. Set appropriate goals for the program. Present funding options to management. Make decisions about fee assessment for program participation. Develop budgeting proposal for management.

Consider an integrated approach to management. Present your program proposal to management. Develop a break-even analysis. Conceive a plan for health screening. Develop plans to guarantee employee safety during program participation. Build evaluation mechanisms into the program.

**Implementation**

Develop a marketing strategy based on the 4 Ps of marketing. Develop ideas for promoting the program. Consider ways to promote program adherence and ways to attract nonparticipants and high-risk employees.

Conceive end-of-program rewards. Develop a health fair. Conceive ways to recruit employees to participate in the fair.

**Evaluation**

Review program goals and objectives. Establish a time frame, measurement intervals, and compatible evaluation design.

Perform measurements and provide feedback to employees and management.

If appropriate, conduct an economic evaluation, such as a benefit-cost analysis or cost-effectiveness analysis.

**Figure 1**  The WHP program planning framework.

Part IV contains the final two chapters of the book, dealing with other considerations in WHP. Chapter 9 presents an overview of various factors confronting small and multisite businesses in trying to incorporate WHP. Chapter 10, written mainly for students, presents practical information on how to academically and professionally prepare for a career in the broad field of WHP. The chapter offers tips on selecting a strong academic curriculum as well as preparing for an internship and honing your skills for a job interview.

## WHAT'S NEW IN THIS EDITION

New features added to this edition of *Worksite Health Promotion* include learning objectives for each chapter and an updated listing of key resources. New sections cover

- tailoring WHP programs around an organization's mission and vision,
- e-health management communication tools,
- using the stages of change framework with programming incentives,
- exploring the relationship between employee health and productivity, and
- using three tiers of evaluation.

These new features are added for readers to consider using in their new and expanding WHP programming efforts.

WHP has strong potential as an effective health and productivity management tool. The text that follows will enhance your personal and professional efforts in this dynamic, ever-changing field.

# Acknowledgments

In the 7 years since I wrote my last book on worksite health promotion, many of America's finest WHP program directors and managers have generously shared information with me in hopes that others could benefit from their expertise. Their ideas and strategies on screening, programming, marketing, and evaluation have given me a good perspective of the daily challenges confronting these visionary, hard-working individuals. I thank each of you for your valued contributions. I also owe many thanks to all of the WHP professionals who have graciously provided preinternship and internship opportunities to our WHP student majors over the years. Finally, a big thank you to my colleagues at ECU for supporting the creation of an undergraduate WHP program which, in part, has given me an opportunity to write this book.

# Initiating Worksite Health Promotion

# The Case for Worksite Health Promotion

After reading this chapter you will be able to

→ Describe the major factors responsible for medical care inflation and how rising health care costs directly affect employers.

→ Describe several significant events that characterize the history of worksite health promotion.

→ List various factors that motivate organizations to establish worksite health promotion programs.

→ Describe the relationship between health risk status and medical care expenses.

**W**hat is the future of business? A day rarely passes that we don't hear of another layoff, labor strike, corporate takeover, bankruptcy, or plant closing. However, the rising cost of paying for employees' health care is an even greater problem for most employers. In America, the business portion of the nation's total health care bill increased from 18% in 1965 to more than 40% in 2006. Moreover, many companies report that the annual cost of providing employee health benefits has reached approximately 50% of their business profits. Perhaps the most glaring example of today's health care cost problem is reflected in a study by the Lewin Group. It showed that the following occurred over a 4-year period:

1. Average individual wages increased 12.4% while employee health care insurance premiums increased nearly 36%.

2. In 26 states employee health care insurance premiums rose over 40%.

3. On average employer-paid premiums increased 32%.

4. The number of Americans who had personal health care costs exceeding 25% of earnings rose from 11.6 million to 14.3 million, or about 1 of every 10 working adults.

Worldwide, health care cost inflation continues to rise several times faster than general inflation (consumer price index) because many forces—demographic, economic, philosophical, cultural, political, social, and administrative—exert tremendous influence in the global economy. Collectively, these forces have driven annual health care cost increases above the annual growth of the **gross domestic product** (or GDP, the total dollar value of all goods and services produced annually by businesses and industries within a country). To better understand the economic realities of this phenomenon, consider the significant percentage growth of America's health care tab as a percentage of its GDP over the past three decades and the projected increase in the next decade (see figure 1.1). Note that the percentage of the GDP tied to health care costs has risen from less than 10% in the 1970s

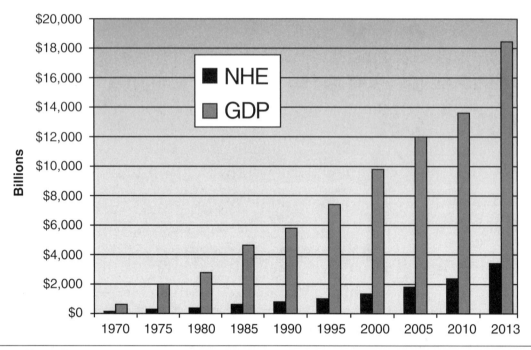

**Figure 1.1**  National health care expenditures (NHE) compared to the gross domestic product (GDP) in the United States.

to 15% in 2006 and is expected to exceed 18% by 2013. Yet, many countries throughout the world also spend a sizable portion of their financial assets on health care (see figure 1.2). Ironically, nations that spend the highest percentage of their GDP on health care do not necessarily have the longest disability-free lifespans (see table 1.1). Specifically, this is defined as the average level of population health as reported in terms of disability-adjusted life expectancy (DALE). DALE is most easily understood as the expectation of life lived in equivalent full health.

In the 1980s and 1990s, health care economists blamed about 85% of the health care cost spiral on economic forces such as medical inflation, new technological advances, more regulatory compliance, and cost shifting (when health care providers shift a portion of unpaid bills to insured employers and employees). The remaining 15% of the cost spiral was attributed to rising demand or utilization. However, in the past decade, because life expectancy has increased, utilization factors have virtually equaled the direct impact of economic factors on today's rising health care tab. This is particularly true in developing nations because greater life expectancy rates correspond with rising health care costs.

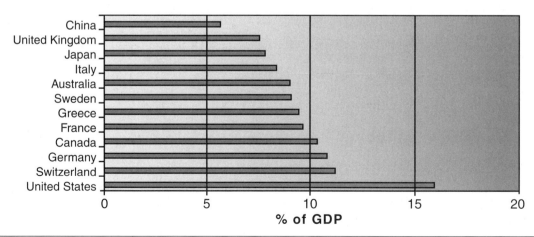

**Figure 1.2**  National health care expenditures (NHE) expressed as percentage of the gross domestic product (GDP) in selected countries.

**Table 1.1  DALE in Selected Countries by Ranking in the World Health Organization (WHO)**

| WHO rank | Nation | DALE at birth |
|----------|--------|---------------|
| 1 | Japan | 74.5 |
| 2 | Australia | 73.2 |
| 3 | France | 73.1 |
| 4 | Sweden | 73.0 |
| 6 | Italy | 72.7 |
| 7 | Greece | 72.5 |
| 8 | Switzerland | 72.5 |
| 12 | Canada | 72.0 |
| 14 | United Kingdom | 71.7 |
| 22 | Germany | 70.4 |
| 24 | United States | 70.0 |
| 82 | China | 62.3 |

Because employers typically pay a higher percentage of a nation's health care tab than any other payer, businesses and industries are naturally concerned about today's rising medical costs and what, if anything, they can do to contain this growing liability. Because increased demand and other utilization factors are driving a substantial portion of their costs, in the past decade many employers have implemented a host of cost-containment strategies, including worksite health promotion (WHP) programs. The overriding premise for establishing WHP programs lies in the assumption that such interventions will (1) reduce modifiable risk factors, which will thereby (2) improve a person's overall health status, which, in turn, will (3) reduce their demand for health care. This premise will be explored later in the chapter.

# A BRIEF HISTORY OF WORKSITE HEALTH PROMOTION

What does worksite health promotion mean to you? The Report of the 2000 Joint Committee on Health Education Terminology (18 professionals representing the professional societies in the Coalition of National Health Education Organizations and various federal agencies) defined worksite health promotion (WHP) as "A combination of educational, organizational, and environmental activities designed to improve the health and safety of employees and their families" (Report of the 2000 Joint Committee on Health Education Terminology, p. 10).

One of the first worksite-based recreation and fitness programs for employees evolved over a century ago in 1879 when the Pullman Company formed its own athletic association. Five years later, John R. Patterson, president of National Cash Register (NCR Corporation), regularly assembled his employees at dawn for prework horseback rides. In 1894, he instituted morning and afternoon exercise breaks and, a decade later, built an employee gym. To top it off, in 1911 he added a 325-acre recreation park for employees. Around this time, Sears, Roebuck and Company also promoted healthy lifestyles to its retail workers.

In the 1930s, when the nation was recovering from the Great Depression, Milton Hershey (Hershey Foods Corporation) built an impressive employee recreation complex that included an indoor swimming pool. The pool surface was built with tile that Mr. Hershey purchased in Argentina while buying cocoa beans for his chocolate.

The growth of worksite recreation and fitness programs appeared to level off for a decade until the National Employee Services and Recreation Association (NESRA; now Employee Services Management [ESM] Association) was formed in 1941 and spearheaded greater interest in employee recreation programs. In 1953, Texas Instruments drafted the initial constitution and bylaws for its employee recreation program and, a decade later, established a half-million-dollar, 8-acre recreational center for Dallas-area employees and their families. In the early 1950s, Sweden-based Scania corporation established a comprehensive support system in various departments offering health education, skill-building courses, and support to the daily line operations and over 700 managers for them to make healthier lifestyle choices. In the late 1950s, PepsiCo established its physical fitness program, which eventually grew into an industry leader in the 1980s. In the early 1960s, Sentry Insurance creatively established its fitness program in the basement coal bunker at its headquarters in Stevens Point, Wisconsin. Rockwell International and Xerox Corporation also established their well-known fitness programs in the 1960s. In 1968, American Can and NASA initiated employee fitness programs; the latter organization was one of the first worksites to publish its program evaluation findings in 1972.

The ESM Association estimates that over 50,000 organizations exist with on-site fitness programs, and nearly 1,000 of them employ full-time program directors.

Although the bulk of WHP efforts centered on recreation and physical fitness through the first half of the 20th century, the advent of Employee Assistance Programs (EAPs) became evident in several larger worksites in the 1950s. Currently, more than 10,000 companies have EAPs, which were initially designed to help employees with alcohol problems. However, the scope of EAPs was broadly expanded throughout the 1970s to offer all employees a wide menu of services that included stress management, flexible work accommodations, eldercare assistance, family care spending accounts, personal counseling, preretirement planning, financial planning, and so on. Some companies have integrated their EAP services within a broader Quality of Work Life (QWL) program to administratively simplify their operations as well as create a more cost-effective approach.

In 1970, the Occupational Safety and Health Act (OSHA) was created in the United States to literally clean up and regulate the worksite environment and instill safer work practices in American worksites. In addition, the Act was effective in raising employers' awareness of employees' health and probably gave some companies an impetus to expand their safety programs into a comprehensive safety and WHP program. Two years later, Japan's Industrial Safety and Health Law and related ordinances were enacted. The law is largely responsible for the significant decline in the number of serious occupational injuries over the past 50 years. Moreover, the law stipulates that health promotion is an employer's obligation.

In 1976, Osaka Gas Company in Japan set up a health care system that has improved the health and physical fitness capabilities of its employees over the past 30 years. A year later, Kimberly-Clark Corporation built a $2.5 million, state-of-the-art health management complex for employees and retirees in Neenah, Wisconsin. Two years later, Mesa Petroleum built a $2.5 million, 30,000 square-foot, on-site fitness center that serves as the centerpiece for employee health screenings and various health promotion programs.

In the 1980s, more WHP programs expanded beyond their traditional fitness center approach and incorporated a holistic menu of wellness programs such as stress management, low-back care, smoking cessation, nutrition, prenatal health, weight control, annual health fairs, and weekly lunchtime learning sessions. A decade later, as the era of personal responsibility and self-development evolved at many worksites, WHP expanded into the arenas of medical self-care, post-pregnancy accommodations (e.g., lactation rooms), ergonomic assessments, and exercise courses such as body shaping, kick-boxing, spinning, and self-defense or martial arts.

Surveys conducted by the Japanese Ministry of Labour of over 12,000 private worksites employing 10 or more workers showed periodic health exams were conducted at nearly 90% of the locations; nearly 45% offered WHP activities. Of these worksites, 48% had sporting events, 46% had exercise programs, and 35% had health counseling.

More Canadian worksites embraced WHP in the late 1990s. Employers offering at least one wellness initiative increased from 44% in 1996 to 64% in 2000. One survey showed that nearly 50% of responding Canadian worksites offered EAP programs, 48% offered first aid and CPR training, 36% offered smoking cessation programs, and 33% provided ergonomics training.

As the 21st century approached, a growing number of worksites became aware of the evolving research on the correlation between a person's health status, lifestyle, and productivity. Although most of the initial health and productivity management (HPM) interventions were adopted in larger worksites, some surveys suggest that HPM will continue to grow in both large and mid-sized companies over the next decade. Concomitantly, some WHP industry observers expect more companies to adopt integrated health management (IHM) networks to enable various departments and divisions to work more effectively together in reaching their employees in a cost-effective manner.

Currently, only 50% of all American worksites with more than 750 employees provide some type of WHP programs to their employees. Smaller worksites are even less likely to offer such programs. For example, WHP programs are found in only 38% of worksites employing 250 to 749 employees; and in just 33% for those employing fewer than 49 persons. Yet, Healthy People 2010

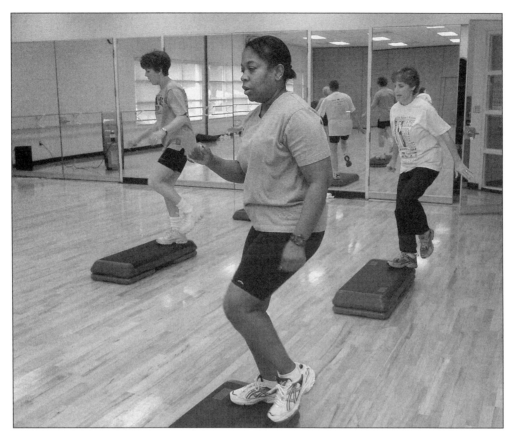

Objective 7-5 of the Healthy People 2010 report states: "Increase to at least 75% the proportion of workplaces that offer a comprehensive health promotion program to their employees." (Healthy People 2010, pp. 7-18)

recommends that many more worksites should provide such programs and that future programs should be comprehensive in nature, not just offer a single intervention.

WHP historians cite fundamental differences behind WHP initiatives in the United States, Japan, and Europe. For example, legislation was a driving force in Japan but not in the United States or Europe. WHP essentially emerged in Japan against the backdrop of fears in the government concerning low productivity because of the rising number of older workers. In contrast, much of the WHP initiative in the United States was driven by rising employee health care costs, and in Europe amid fears surrounding work ability. Specifically, the major factors affecting workers' health were thought to be their personal lifestyles in the United States and Japan and organizational factors in Europe. Consequently, WHP in the United States and Japan emphasized intervention in personal lifestyles, while in Europe the focus was on organization and the workplace environment.

# WHY BUSINESSES OFFER WORKSITE HEALTH PROMOTION

Treating one's employees and fellow workers with respect and care is not just the right thing to do, it is also good business. Based on several surveys, the most common reasons given for establishing WHP interventions are reportedly to (1) attract and retain good employees, (2) keep workers healthy, (3) improve employee morale, (4) improve employee productivity, and (5) reduce employee health care costs. Some of the underlying justification for these reasons is as follows:

• *Absenteeism*. Because one half of all unscheduled absences in the United States are attributed to minor ailments that are tied to potentially modifiable behaviors, more companies are offering specific types of WHP programs and wellness incentives to their employees. It is interesting that absenteeism and presenteeism (being at work but not performing up to par) are reportedly more compelling reasons for many European companies to initiate WHP initiatives than health care costs.

• *Accessibility*. The workplace is usually a good setting in which to offer educational and motivational programs to many people at one time.

• *Aging workforce*. Every 8 seconds, another baby boomer turns 50. As American workers age and experience more health problems, many employers are using age-appropriate interventions to slow the effects of the aging process and detect problems earlier.

• *Business contacts*. Health promotion events such as community health fairs and corporate challenge events create new business contacts.

• *Competition*. Concern about retaining valuable employees is prompting companies to provide financial incentives and other perks to enhance morale and increase retention.

• *Growing interest*. Interest in personal health enhancement and health care cost containment is reflected in today's print and electronic media coverage.

• *Health insurance premiums*. Employer-paid health insurance premiums for employees and dependents have doubled in the past decade and, thus, jeopardize an organization's net profits.

• *Image*. Many corporate leaders realize that successful WHP programs can boost a company's image among workers, community, and industry peers.

• *Productivity*. Because healthy employees generally outperform unhealthy employees, more companies are offering health promotion programs to achieve greater HPM outcomes.

• *Workers' compensation costs*. Up to one half of all workers' compensation claims involve musculoskeletal strains and sprains. Because the vast majority of strain- and sprain-related injuries are tied to poor fitness levels, numerous worksites are integrating workers' comp–related case management, work hardening, and return-to-work protocols into a WHP programming framework.

But does WHP actually address all these concerns effectively? Let's look at some data that may help answer that question.

# FACTORS BEHIND RISING HEALTH CARE COSTS

Some would argue that WHP is not effective in containing, much less reducing, a business' health care costs because many factors in addition to employee health—or lack of it—have contributed to the rapid rise in health care costs.

## Economic Factors

As is true with any product or service in the market, health care costs fluctuate depending on such factors as inflation, overhead, and operating expenses. When the service is providing medical or health care, some of the expenses necessary for continued operation (e.g., insurance or cost of materials) are much greater than they are for other services, and that expense is passed on at least in part to the consumer. If a company offers to its employees the benefit of health insurance, it is the company rather than the individual that takes on all or part of the financial burden passed on by the providing health care agency when the agency's costs escalate. Many companies that absorb this ever-increasing expense must look for ways to cut the costs if they are going to remain in operation. Consequently, companies are becoming more interested in the causes of rising health care costs as they seek possible ways to manipulate the causes in order to contain costs. Let's look at some of the major forces driving today's health care inflation.

• Inflation is a driving force as the medical care services component of the Consumer Price Index (a measure of inflation based on the price of a group of commonly purchased goods and services such as groceries and electricity) often rises two to three times as fast as other items in the index. Yet, some health economists argue that high costs are necessary if we are to improve our medical care systems.

• Cost shifting adds one fourth to one third more cost to the average health care bill. Cost shifting is the "hidden tax" that doctors and hospitals shift to employers and paying customers to compensate for patients who cannot or do not pay their bills.

• New technology leads to innovative but costly treatments. Today, many illnesses can be diagnosed but not necessarily cured. Although maintenance programs and life-support systems may keep patients alive for long periods, these heroic interventions carry a huge price tag. Despite the huge price tag, many people still believe that technology is essential for improved health and longevity.

• Catastrophic cases involving, for example, transplant operations, HIV/AIDS, kidney dialysis, and premature infants with complications consume a lot of health care resources.

• The high cost of malpractice insurance for doctors and hospitals is passed on to paying patients and their employers. This is a secondary type of cost shifting.

• In today's litigious society, more doctors and hospitals practice what is known as defensive medicine—doing more procedures than necessary, for example—in an effort to protect themselves from potential lawsuits.

## Demographic Shifts

Four changes in the makeup of the global workforce are having drastic effects on individual health status and health care concerns. These shifts affect not only physical health, but mental health costs as well. They are

1. the aging of the workforce,
2. the entry of more women into the workplace,
3. the rising proportion of people of color working in many countries, and
4. the growing number of people who have to work two jobs to make ends meet.

These changes are particularly notable in North American, European, and Asian countries. For example, as more people live longer and use more health care services, the overall volume of health care services will continue to grow. One of the most important factors shaping the United States is the aging of Americans. In fact, the post–World War II baby boom that produced today's 27- to 45-year-olds is not about babies; it's about the growing percentage of older workers and their future impact on America's worksites and corporate health care costs. For example, middle-aged workers (35- to 54-year-olds) currently make up more than 50% of America's workforce. In contrast, younger, entry-level workers—especially in the 16- to 34-year-old age group—comprise just one third of today's workforce.

Eldercare is one of the fastest-growing needs of many workers. Currently, out of some 35 million adult Americans over 65, about 8.0 million need some form of long-term care. Of those, 1.7 million are in nursing homes. The remaining 6.3 million are getting some kind of home care within or outside the health care system. Yet, fewer than one third of all companies surveyed provide their employees with eldercare assistance benefits.

The realization that the mental health of its employees can significantly influence a company's bottom line has caused an increasing number of employers to take a serious look at issues raised by the demographic shifts just listed. Although some older workers can outperform their younger coworkers through greater efficiency, as a group they still encounter greater scrutiny and discrimination from managers and younger workers who often do not understand the aging process and do not appreciate that older workers can be productive in their later years.

Since 1980, the Hispanic American population has grown more than 50% while the African American population has grown more than 20%, greatly outpacing the 10% growth of Caucasians. This trend has resulted in more Hispanic Americans and African Americans in the workforce, a disproportionate number of whom work in the fast-growing, but lower-paying service sector of the economy. Women are also entering the American workforce at an unprecedented rate and comprise about 60% of the labor force. Ironically, these demographic shifts are occurring throughout many parts of the world. For example, Japan is becoming one of the oldest societies in the industrialized world; a number of European countries (Germany, in particular) have rapidly aging populations that are more pronounced than in the United States; Latin America, the Middle East, and some Asian countries, on the other hand, are currently experiencing major population growth. Undoubtedly, these shifts are creating greater stress on working men and women to successfully balance family life and work life. Consequently, employers have a greater responsibility to provide EAPs and QWL programs for their employees.

## Major Employee Health Risks

Despite having a slightly longer lifespan than a decade ago, the average American's health status has not improved. In fact, more women are smoking than ever before and therefore face a greater risk of heart disease, lung cancer, and other smoking-related ailments. And, despite the plethora of fat-free foods and exercise options in today's marketplace, more than 60% of American adults are overweight or obese. According to the findings from a survey of 400 business leaders, various risk factors negatively impact employees' health status. For example, the most common risk factors, as ranked by the business leaders in order of frequency, were:

1. Excess stress
2. High blood pressure
3. Cigarette smoking
4. Back injuries
5. Overweight
6. Alcohol abuse
7. High blood cholesterol
8. Drug abuse
9. Depression
10. Other mental health problems

Independent studies conducted at Bank One, Ceridian Corporation, Dow Chemical, DuPont, Daimler/Chrysler, General Electric, General Motors, Goldman Sachs, Osaka Gas, Procter & Gamble, Prudential Insurance, Scania, and Steelcase indicate that most of the identified risk factors are due, in varying degrees, to individual lifestyles. (Goetzel et al., 1998; Kirsten, 2005; and Milliman & Roberson, Inc., 1995).

## COST SHARING

As many corporate benefit managers can attest, lower health care utilization rates don't necessarily result in lower corporate health care expenses. Why? Because many of the forces that drive today's health care costs—cost shifting, medical inflation, new technology, and other economic forces—are influenced primarily by market forces, not by an employer's actions.

The time is coming—some say it is here—when the availability and cost of specific health care benefits will depend on an employee's lifestyle and risk level. Consequently, some observers speculate that WHP programs may no longer be offered primarily as a fringe benefit, but as an economic necessity—for the primary purpose of helping high-risk and unhealthy employees reduce their risk factors in order to qualify for health insurance.

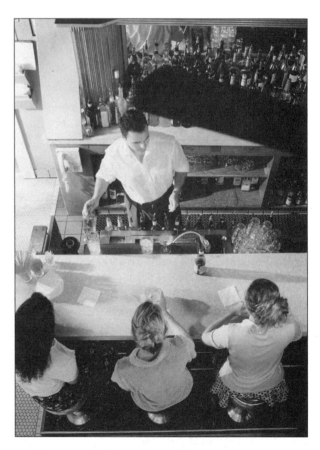

An ongoing debate exists about whether lifestyle-related claims such as smoking-induced lung diseases and alcohol-induced motor vehicle accidents—claims directly tied to a person's choice—should be covered by company-paid health insurance.

In a 2003 nationwide poll of chief executive officers (CEOs) in the United States, health care costs was the most pressing cost issue (43%) followed by litigation (20%) and energy prices (19%). In 2004, the Society of Human Resource Management conducted a survey in which 247 of the Fortune 500 corporations answered this question: "Do corporations have a responsibility to promote the health and wellness of their employees?" More than 80% of the respondents said yes. (*Employee Benefit News*, 2005).

In another nationwide poll of 1,500 U.S. CEOs, 90% of the respondents ranked rising health insurance premium costs as their greatest cost concern. When asked how they would contain future health care costs, respondents overwhelmingly (80%) said **cost sharing** was the preferred method. In fact, over half of the respondents thought cost sharing was effective in controlling health care expenses. Many employers feel that a moderate cost-sharing arrangement ($350 deductible and 10% co-payment, for example) can produce substantial cost savings without discouraging necessary medical care. Yet, some health care economists contend that cost sharing does very little, if anything, to reduce health care inflation because it merely shifts the cost from employers to employees. In reality, they argue, cost sharing causes some people to delay seeking treatment when they really need it. Such delays could lead to needless suffering, worsening of an existing health problem, and resulting in even higher health care costs. Although these arguments sound reasonable, no conclusive evidence shows that the average cost-sharing arrangement ($500 family deductible and a 15% co-payment) causes insured individuals who really need health care to postpone treatment.

## HEALTH COSTS AND HEALTH PROMOTION

Considering the high percentage of unhealthy workers, what kind of impact should employers expect from their health promotion efforts? Independent studies conducted on employees at numerous worksites indicate the following:

• More than 50% of corporate health care costs come from potentially modifiable (lifestyle) risk factors such as poor diet, tobacco use, physical inactivity, and obesity.

• Potentially modifiable risk factors such as smoking, physical inactivity, and obesity contribute to significantly higher short-term health care expenses.

• Persons with high-risk profiles generally have higher health care costs than persons with low-risk profiles (see figure 1.3).

In particular, a study of 6,000 Chrysler Corporation employees over a period of 3 years showed a strong relationship between an individual's risk level and health care usage. Ten factors were studied including smoking, body weight, exercise, alcohol use, driving habits, eating habits, stress, mental health, cholesterol, and blood pressure. For example, smokers had 31% higher annual claim costs than nonsmokers; persons with an elevated risk for obesity used hospitals 143% more than their low-risk peers; and persons with a poor diet had 41% higher medical costs than those with a good diet.

Numerous worksites have reported cost savings tied to their respective WHP programs. A sampling of their cost-saving outcomes follows:

• **Aetna:** Five state-of-the-art fitness centers keep exercisers' health care costs nearly $300 lower than nonexercisers.

• **British Columbia Hydro:** The company's WHP program generates a 3:1 benefit-to-cost ratio.

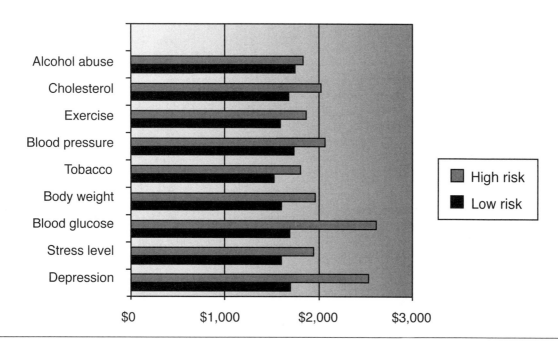

**Figure 1.3** Differences in mean annual medical expenditures for high-risk versus low-risk employees.

• **Canada Life Insurance:** The company's fitness program generated a benefit-to-cost ratio of 3.43:1 in 1 year.

• **City of Birmingham, Alabama:** Health risk appraisal screenings and customized interventions save the city approximately $1 million in annual medical care expenses.

• **L.L. Bean:** Annual health insurance premiums are half the national average because of a healthy workforce.

• **Coors Brewing Company:** The company saves more than $600,000 a year from its on-site fitness, cardiac rehabilitation, and recreation programs.

• **Johnson & Johnson:** Customized health screening saves $13 million a year in less absenteeism and health care usage.

• **Osaka Gas Company:** The company's WHP program has increased productivity and morale while decreasing smoking rates and premature mortality among employees.

• **The Quaker Oats Company:** Health insurance premiums are about one third less than the national average because of its integrated health management approach.

• **Steelcase:** Personal health counselors motivate high-risk employees to reduce major risk factors, generating an estimated $20 million over 10 years.

• **Tenneco Corporation:** Acute health care costs dropped 43% after implementing a WHP program that features a state-of-the-art fitness center and customized health education offerings.

• **Union Pacific Railroad:** This company saves more than $3 million annually in hypertension- and smoking-related costs. In 1990, nearly 33% of UPR's total medical care costs were lifestyle related; by 2001, only 18.8% were related to lifestyle.

Despite these impressive statistics, health promotion is only part of the equation in building a comprehensive health management framework that will create a healthier and more productive workforce (see figure 1.4). In essence, an organization's ability to achieve this goal depends largely on whether it can simultaneously do the following:

• Influence employees and dependents to be responsible users of health care services.

• Provide appropriate health care benefits to employees and dependents.

• Motivate employees and dependents to use only quality-focused, cost-conscious health care providers.

• Analyze health care claims data on a regular basis, and use the results to determine appropriate health management initiatives.

• Provide a comprehensive WHP program to meet the needs of all employees.

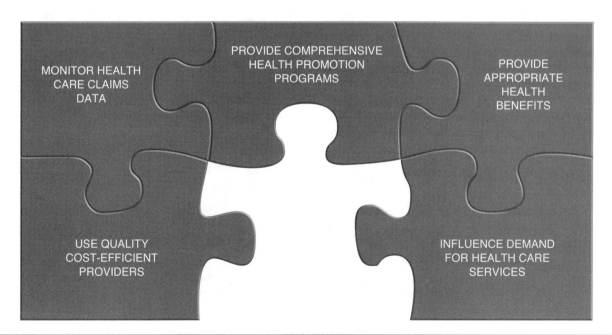

**Figure 1.4** Key corporate cost-containment strategies that comprise a comprehensive health management framework.

As shown in figure 1.5, in order to reach these desirable goals, health promotion and health care cost management efforts must appeal to and reach as many employees as possible through three levels of effort:

1. primary prevention,
2. secondary prevention, and
3. tertiary care.

The odds for developing a healthy workforce and worksite will depend on how well employers use their resources in building and maintaining an effective WHP program. Chapter 2 also describes basic principles to consider when designing a program.

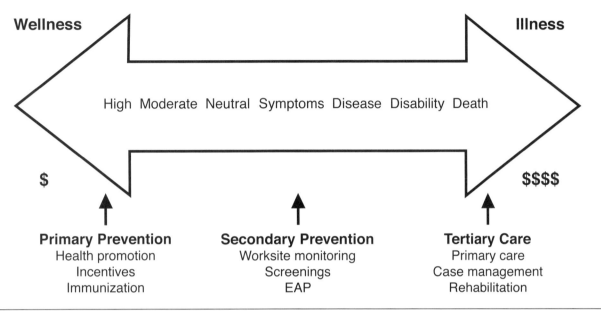

**Figure 1.5**  Examples of primary prevention, secondary prevention, and tertiary care interventions relevant to various stages of health status and their correlation to corporate medical care expenses.

## WHAT WOULD YOU DO?

While the growth in WHP programs since the early 1980s has been impressive, many programs lack comprehensive offerings or sufficient length to impact employee health status and work performance. Some WHP industry leaders contend that the future growth of WHP programs as well as their impact on health and productivity will largely be determined by how WHP personnel deal with the following factors:

→ Positioning WHP efforts to make a dual health promotion and cost-containment impact.

→ Incorporating more rigorous evaluation of WHP efforts to improve their programming efforts.

→ Some workers viewing WHP programs as intrusive and invasive to privacy.

→ The perception that successful WHP programs will increase the retired population that receives Social Security and Medicare and employer-paid health insurance—which, consequently, may actually produce net costs to employers and society.

→ Expanding the scope of WHP programs to help dependents, especially those who have mental health problems because a disproportionately large share of corporate health care costs are tied to dependents and mental health conditions.

→ Dealing with the fact that WHP program costs are immediate and continuous compared with risk reduction and economic benefits that may not occur for months or years.

➜ Motivating at-risk employees and dependents who often rely on their company-subsidized health insurance benefits to treat their ailments rather than participate in WHP programs as a preventive measure.

In your view, which of the preceding factors is most challenging for WHP professionals? Why? What additional factors do you think will challenge the future success of WHP?

# Determining Employees' Needs and Interests

After reading this chapter you will be able to

→ Develop an awareness of several strategies that can be used to identify organizational and employee health needs.

→ Distinguish between needs identification tools and interest assessment tools.

→ Identify several precautions when using health risk appraisal instruments.

→ Describe how to compare identified needs against employee interests in order to develop an appropriate plan of action.

Considering such pressures of downsizing, global competition, and rising production costs, every facet of a business today is being scrutinized by upper management. Because it may be a relatively new endeavor for many businesses, worksite health promotion must be planned and positioned even more carefully than other business strategies. Thus, it is important to accurately determine employees' needs and interests because this stage is the initiation stage of planning WHP programs.

Identification essentially deals with the needs of the workforce, whereas assessment focuses on the desires and intentions of employees and on available resources for approaching problems recognized during identification.

## IDENTIFYING EMPLOYEES' NEEDS

Identification begins with forming a task force to identify a company's demographics (i.e., age and ethnicity distribution, ratio of females to males, education levels, and so on), the existing and potential health-related problems of its workforce, and employee interest in participating in programs to improve their health and well-being.

## Forming a Task Force

The fate of a WHP program depends largely on management's philosophy toward employee health issues. When management personnel lead healthy lifestyles themselves, they are more inclined to support health enhancement activities at the worksite. This inclination also depends on whether they see strong employee interest in the activities. An effective way to spark employee interest is to involve them in planning and implementing the program. Such involvement gives employees a sense of ownership of the program and greatly increases the chances that they will commit to it.

Although at small worksites the site manager or a supervisor might personally solicit input on employee needs and interests, this personalized approach is usually not practical for larger organizations. For larger businesses, the first step in planning a successful WHP program is to form a Health Management Task Force (HMTF) consisting of management and employee representatives. For maximum representation, the task force should include representatives from every department or job classification. In unionized worksites, it's important to include union representatives as well. Although the percentage of union workers has dropped substantially since the 1980s, unions remain a dynamic force in many worksites and can enhance WHP efforts by encouraging employee participation and working closely with management.

Other key issues to consider in organizing an HMTF include:

- Eligibility criteria used to select, appoint, or elect members
- Length of term served by HMTF members
- Number or percentage of management and nonmanagement members serving on the HMTF

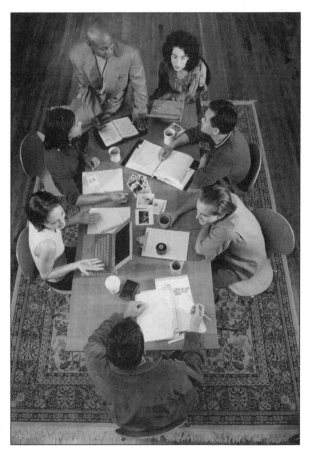

In all worksite settings, the HMTF needs a leader who is respected by employees and managers, skilled in working with small and large groups, sincerely interested in employee health issues, and able to be objective so that the task force is fair to all parties.

- Frequency of scheduled meetings (e.g., weekly, bi-monthly, monthly)
- To whom the HMTF reports
- Defining the primary role of HMTF (e.g., planning, implementing, and so on)
- Determining the level of influence of HMTF (e.g., advisory only, policy making, and so on)
- Recognition of or compensation for service (e.g., release time from job, overtime pay if duties performed beyond normal work hours, and so on)

Once a task force and its leaders have been secured, the next steps are to identify health-related problems at the worksite and to evaluate overall interest in programs that WHP might offer.

## Identifying Health-Related Problems

Because employees' health needs and interests vary from worksite to worksite, the HMTF should carefully assess each workforce for specific problems. For example, is the number of low-back injuries high enough to justify a back injury prevention program? How big a problem is smoking at the worksite? Is the worksite culture conducive to personal health promotion opportunities? What are the best days and times to offer particular programs? Will employees resist the programs unless they have a financial incentive? These are just a few questions that the task force should consider.

An early responsibility for the HMTF is to solicit input from workers at all job levels to ensure that employee needs and interests are accurately identified. Identification strategies should include analyzing

- workforce demographic data,
- employee health records,
- health care claims and costs,
- workers' compensation claims and cost data,
- worksite environment, and
- health risk appraisal data.

Appendix A highlights a Personal Health Questionnaire that you can distribute to employers to gather more information during the identification phase.

The minimum demographic data to acquire include the ratio of male-to-female, salaried-to-hourly, and day-to-night workers; age groups; ethnicity; and the percentage of workers with dependents. This information will be key in planning the types of programs that will be the most useful and appropriate for WHP.

Because of the need to protect each employee's medical privacy and health status, employee health records should be accessed and reviewed only by authorized personnel. In many cases, this information can be used to compile a group health data sheet, listing the most prevalent health problems. A sample data sheet is shown in table 2.1.

The availability and specificity of health care claims and cost data vary greatly from worksite to worksite. The data may be handled by a specific department or, in other cases, an employer may need to ask its insurer or third-party administrator to provide these data. Table 2.2 shows claims

and costs by major diagnostic category (MDC) and subcategories, which are identified by either a diagnostic-related group (DRG) as shown in table 2.3 or international classification of disease

### Table 2.1   Sample Group Health Data Sheet for a Workforce of 200 Employees

| Health condition | Number | Percentage |
|---|---|---|
| Overweight or obese | 65 | 32.5% |
| Smoke cigarettes | 52 | 26.0% |
| High blood pressure | 48 | 24.0% |
| Joint injury | 18 | 9.0% |
| Chronic bronchitis | 17 | 8.5% |
| Low-back pain | 16 | 8.0% |
| High blood cholesterol | 15 | 7.5% |
| Hearing loss, one ear | 10 | 5.0% |

### Table 2.2   Sample Listing of Major Diagnostic Categories (MDCs)

| # of MDC | # of claims | Total charges | Charge per claim |
|---|---|---|---|
| 01 Infectious | 2 | $948 | $474 |
| 02 Neoplasm | 5 | $58,924 | $11,784 |
| 03 Endocrine, nutrition, and metabolic | 4 | $1,880 | $470 |
| 04 Blood | 0 | $0 | $0 |
| 05a Mental | 10 | $8,900 | $890 |
| 05b Alcohol/Drug | 7 | $5,180 | $740 |
| 06 Nervous | 2 | $1,960 | $980 |
| 07 Circulatory | 3 | $13,500 | $4,500 |
| 08 Respiratory | 3 | $1,050 | $350 |
| 09 Digestive | 4 | $1,808 | $452 |
| 10 Genitourinary | 17 | $6,613 | $389 |
| 11a Pregnancy | 2 | $6,440 | $3,230 |
| 11b Newborn | 2 | $2,220 | $1,110 |
| 11c Perinatal | 1 | $1,890 | $1,890 |
| 12 Skin/subcutaneous | 7 | $1,575 | $225 |
| 13 Musculoskeletal | 14 | $7,840 | $560 |
| 14 Congenital | 0 | $0 | $0 |
| 15 Signs/Symptoms/Ill-defined | 47 | $3,150 | $225 |
| 16 Accident/Injury/Poisoning | 4 | $1,504 | $376 |
| 17 Other, ill-defined | 8 | $3,192 | $399 |

**Table 2.3  Sample Listing of Diagnostic-Related Group (DRG) Claims Within Selected Major Diagnostic Categories (MDCs)**

| MDC DRG # | # claims | Total charges | Average charge |
|---|---|---|---|
| CIRCULATORY | | | |
| 107 Coronary bypass with cardiac catheterization | 3 | $170,506 | $56,835 |
| 138 Cardiac arrhythmia | 1 | $5,240 | $5,240 |
| 143 Chest pain | 7 | $40,474 | $5,782 |
| MENTAL | | | |
| 426 Depressive neuroses | 12 | $9,016 | $751 |
| 430 Psychoses | 27 | $42,061 | $1,557 |
| MUSCULOSKELETAL | | | |
| 216 Biopsy, musculoskeletal tissue | 23 | $112,779 | $4,903 |
| 248 Tendonitis/Bursitis | 6 | $24,832 | $4,138 |
| PREGNANCY | | | |
| 370 Cesarean section with complications | 4 | $24,141 | $6,035 |
| 371 Cesarean section without complications | 70 | $497,000 | $7,100 |
| 373 Vaginal delivery without complications | 81 | $380,628 | $4,699 |
| 389 Full-term neonate with major problems | 2 | $16,326 | $8,163 |

**Table 2.4  Health Care Claim Report Listing of International Classification of Disease (ICD) Claims Within Selected Major Diagnostic Categories (MDCs)**

| # MDC/ICD Code | # of claims | Total charges | Charge per claim |
|---|---|---|---|
| 02 NEOPLASM | | | |
| 172.0 Skin | 2 | $7,192 | $3,596 |
| 174.4 Breast | 1 | $19,484 | $19,484 |
| 183.0 Ovary | 1 | $15,400 | $15,400 |
| 188.3 Bladder | 1 | $16,848 | $16,848 |
| 05A MENTAL | | | |
| 300.0 Anxiety | 4 | $1,927 | $481 |
| 300.4 Depression | 5 | $5,975 | $1,195 |
| 301.3 Explosive personality | 1 | $998 | $998 |
| 07 CIRCULATORY | | | |
| 402.1 Hypertension | 1 | $3,256 | $3,256 |
| 414.0 Atherosclerosis | 1 | $7,777 | $7,777 |
| 455.0 Hemorrhoids | 1 | $2,467 | $2,467 |

(ICD) code (see table 2.4). At a minimum, claims data should include the following:

- Major diagnostic category and associated DRGs or ICDs
- Number of claims and charges per DRG or ICD
- Inpatient versus outpatient claims and charges per DRG or ICD
- Employee-specific versus dependent-specific claims and charges per DRG or ICD

These data will help the task force recognize which WHP programs might be most beneficial and estimate potential savings for the company if a successful WHP program is implemented.

Workers' compensation claims data are typically handled by the medical, safety, risk management, benefits, or human resources department; show the incidence and types of injuries resulting in work-related absence or disability; and indicate any employer-paid compensation paid to injured employees. Like health care claims and costs data, this information helps the task force target programs and is useful in calculating possible savings if a successful WHP program is implemented.

At many worksites, employees can be randomly identified and monitored to determine the prevalence and effect of certain risk factors and work styles on their health status. This is called *climate observation*. For example, employees with certain on-the-job tendencies are more likely to experience specific types of problems as noted in table 2.5.

**Table 2.5  Ailments Commonly Associated with Particular Risk Factors**

| Risk factor | Types of problems |
| --- | --- |
| Sedentary job | Musculoskeletal, circulatory, and mental health |
| Obesity | Musculoskeletal, circulatory, respiratory, and digestive |
| Smoking | Circulatory and respiratory |
| Unhealthy eating | Fatigue-related, circulatory, and digestive |
| Substance abuse | Drug dependence, hyperactivity, apathy, absenteeism, and accidents |
| Low water intake | Urinary tract infections |
| Poor body mechanics | Musculoskeletal |

An environmental checksheet can be used to identify existing and potential problems at a worksite, especially those resulting from working patterns or environmental factors, such as the percentage of time workers are doing physical labor, working at a computer, or performing a repetitive task. Because each worksite and workforce is unique, the sample checksheet in appendix B can be modified to suit particular needs.

## Health Risk Appraisal

One of the most common identification tools used at the worksite is health risk appraisal (HRA). HRA is based on the concept of risk identification, risk assessment, and risk reduction conceived by Dr. Lewis Robbins in 1959. In 1962, Cecelia Conrath, a health educator for the U.S. Cancer Control Program and Dr. William DeMaria of Duke University suggested the term *prospective medicine* for this approach to preventive medicine. Dr. DeMaria defined prospective medicine as "A discipline concerned with the identification of the individual's changing risks of disease and the recognition of his earliest deviations from health" (Society of Prospective Medicine, 1976). It essentially aims to promote health, prevent disease, and thus extend useful life expectancy by complementing the art of medical care with a scientific method, which reduces long-term health risks.

In the early 1960s, the concept of prospective medicine was expanded to include a comprehensive concern for an individual's total—and changing—spectrum of risk factors. Throughout the 1960s and 1970s, as research added to the evolving scientific understanding of risk-factor assessment, appraisal instruments were developed and refined, and they were introduced in public health, university, and worksite settings. Currently, approximately 50 commercialized HRA instruments exist.

HRAs come in a variety of types and price ranges. HRAs can be found in self-scoring formats, computable and scannable questionnaire forms with extensive outcome reports, phone-based tools, and interactive online versions. Some HRAs have added productivity-based questions in the past few years as the issue of health and productivity management has grown in popularity.

It is essential that HRAs be administered in a confidential manner. If HRA results are to be used for individual targeted intervention or incentive programs, consent must be obtained from participants. This requirement may necessitate using a third-party vendor to conduct the HRA to ensure employee confidentiality. In addition, employees need to know that company personnel will not have access to their personal health information.

Despite their widespread appeal, HRAs are not designed to replace physical exams and other screenings performed by a qualified health care provider. Many WHP personnel combine HRAs with biometric screenings because it is a good incentive to boost participation and adds a direct-measure component to the program's planning and evaluation efforts. Common biometric screenings include blood pressure, body composition, cardiovascular fitness, cholesterol (total and HDL), flexibility, glucose, mammography, and physical strength.

Because HRA instruments vary considerably in many features, it is good to review several formats before selecting one for use in a particular setting. Here are some questions to consider before purchasing an HRA:

- Does a single fee cover everything for the HRA; or do separate fees exist for the questionnaire, processing, and printing of reports?
- What discount is available with a bulk order?
- What assurances exist that only authorized personnel will have access to the HRA?
- Does the database reflect a population similar to your workforce?
- What minimum literacy level is required for participants to clearly interpret their HRA results?
- Is a group report (summary) included in the standard package?
- What is the turnaround time?

## Screening for Green

Wellness screening is one of the best ways to assess an organization's health status and target at-risk employees…IF people participate. And perhaps nothing draws participation better than that certain shade of green. Saint Thomas Health Services, a comprehensive health system in Nashville, Tennessee with a staff of more than 3,400, designed a financial incentive screening program that's saving them some serious green. As it turns out, spending money really is one of the best ways to save it.

When the incentive program was first implemented in 1994, 31 percent of Saint Thomas' workforce responded to the $50 incentive applied to their health benefits. Although this was quite a modest response rate, management saw promise in the initiative. They were convinced that raising the amount of the incentive would increase participation.

### A RISKY INVESTMENT?

In the program's second year, a point system was implemented to encourage employees to participate in the health screenings and work toward improving their lifestyles. And this wasn't just any run-of-the-mill incentive program. The Saint Thomas benefits department assembled an award system that gave employees the opportunity to earn up to $300 toward their health benefits if they participated in the wellness screening.

Here's how it works. Individuals earn points based on both behaviors and screening results. Behaviors include participation in the screening, smoking status, and whether or not an individual receives a flu shot. Screening results refer to the actual physical measurements from the screening, such as cholesterol and blood pressure. They can also earn points for showing improvements from their previous screening. First year participants and those participating in non-consecutive years receive only $50. However, those who participate in consecutive years earn anywhere from $100 to $300, depending on their physical measurements.

Improvement points are a key component of the point system—they help motivate employees to change behaviors. For example, an individual with a healthy cholesterol level would receive more points than someone with high cholesterol. But, if someone with high cholesterol reduced their level significantly from the previous year's screening, that person would receive points for the improvement.

### SHOW ME THE MONEY

Even with this enticing system in place, participation rates in 1995 and 1996 were stable at best.

*(continued)*

Then something happened that played in favor of the participants. Congress passed the Health Insurance Portability and Accountability Act (HIPAA). Essentially, this prohibited employers from using health status factors to penalize individuals participating in their health plan. This meant that participants could no longer be given incentives to apply to their health benefits. So, with unsatisfactory participation rates in mind, Saint Thomas made the decision—they would keep the same incentive point system, but give the money directly to participants.

In addition to this unbeatable incentive, Dr. Porr decided that *Wellness: A Choice* would start doing its own advertising in 1997. He wanted to make it impossible not to know about. They used department meetings, elevator posters, payroll stuffers, and direct mail to get the message out to everyone. Plus, the news about free cash obviously traveled fast.

### CASHING IN

It worked. Participation shot up to 44 percent in 1997. Since then, participation has climbed steadily. And, as the popularity for screenings increases, so does the health of many Saint Thomas employees. "Our situation is unique here. Usually, an individual's health risks increase over

time. However, within our employee population, these risk factors have decreased over a seven-year period," Porr says.

By 2001, Saint Thomas' health screening program showed a solid increase in popularity, effectiveness, and bottom line impact. With a participation rate of 52 percent, improved employee health, and an organizational health care cost avoidance of $1.6 million, it's apparent that this company has turned a big incentive into even bigger rewards.

### THE PRACTITIONER BEHIND THE PROGRAM

Denny Porr, PhD, has spent the past 22 years in the administration of private and corporate wellness programs that has taken him across the country as well as overseas. He has developed wellness programs for numerous corporations and hospitals. Denny has also practiced clinical exercise physiology and sports training. Dr. Porr received his Ph.D. from Arizona State University and is currently the Director of Wellness Services overseeing Employee Health Services, Workers' Compensation, the Stress Reduction Program, Nutrition and Food Services, the Wellness Center, and the *Wellness: A Choice* employee wellness screening program at Saint Thomas Hospital in Nashville, Tennessee.

Reprinted, by permission, from Wellness Councils of America, 2002, *Absolute Advantage* (Omaha, NE: WELCO).

# ASSESSING EMPLOYEES' INTERESTS

As the identification process winds down, program planners should move into **assessment,** the second phase of the planning framework. This phase focuses on the desires and intentions of employees and on ways to deal with problems recognized during the identification phase.

## Interest Survey Form

A popular assessment tool is an interest survey form (ISF). In preparing an ISF, program planners should strive to limit it to one page and consider whether a specific or generic format is most appropriate. For example, a generic format, shown on page 22, is a good way to assess employees' interests in various programs and activities. ISFs often include the following:

- Risk-reduction program options (blood pressure, cholesterol, exercise, nutrition, and work–life balance)
- Readiness to change levels (precontemplation, contemplation, preparation, action, and maintenance)
- Program format preferences (seminar, class, self-help, personal coach, Internet or Web-based)
- Participation time preferences (before work, at break time, lunch, or after work)
- Preferred communication channels (e-mail, posters, at-home mailing, staff meeting, and so on)
- Invitation to assist WHP personnel (wellness committee, HMTF, peer support group, and so on)

However, some organizations wish to assess employees' interest in a specific program (exercise, for example) and thus choose to limit the ISF to questions about that program.

To enhance the prospect of getting a high response, employees should be informed of the interest survey form at least twice before they are distributed. Use various delivery channels to publicize and distribute the ISF, such as the following:

- Company newsletter
- Electronic message boards
- E-mail or Web site
- Flyers
- Paycheck stuffers
- Bulletin board displays in key locations

Within a couple of days of publicizing the ISF, the forms should be distributed either personally to each employee or their respective mailbox. When using an e-mail or Internet-based ISF, it's good to publicize the survey 1 or 2 days before its actual distribution to promptly alert respondents and discourage them from deleting the message.

**Table 2.6  Assessing Interest Survey Form (ISF) Feedback**

| Technique | Needs |
|---|---|
| Employee health record | • Elevated BMI (60%)<br>• Previous back injury (30%) |
| Environmental checksheet | • Sedentary job (80%)<br>• Unhealthy snacking (55%) |
| Health risk appraisal | • Poor diet (65%)<br>• High stress (35%) |
| Health claims summary | • Circulatory problems (most expensive)<br>• Low-back injury (most common) |
| ISF | 1. Walking<br>2. Weight loss<br>3. Back health<br>4. Financial planning<br>5. Nutrition |

## Interest Survey

**TELL US WHERE YOU STAND!**

Please check the programs you would like to see offered at our worksite.

| ____ Aerobic exercise | ____ Medical self-care | ____ Stress management |
|---|---|---|
| ____ Back health | ____ Nutrition and diet | ____ Walking |
| ____ Blood pressure control | ____ Prenatal/pregnancy | ____ Weight control |
| ____ First aid and CPR | ____ Quitting smoking | |

Other (list): _____

Would you participate in any of these programs at the worksite on your own time?   Yes____  No____

What days would you prefer?   M____  T____  W____  Th____  F____  Sat____  Sun____

What times would you prefer?   Before work____  At break time____  At lunch____  After work____

What is the biggest barrier for you to overcome in order to participate in a worksite program? _____

_____

Comments_____

_____

_____

Please return this survey to _____ by _____.

Stay tuned for future details!

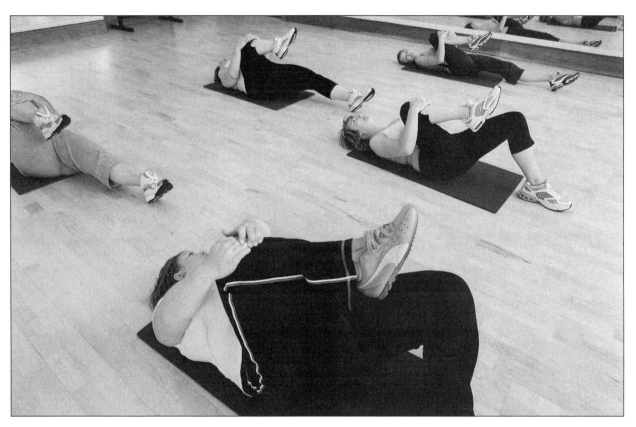

Although a worksite may choose to offer a low-back program independently of other programs, the grid might suggest that better results may be obtained from integrative programming—merging exercise and weight control with the low-back program.

If by the due date for the survey to be returned you have received less than 50% of the forms, you might distribute a reminder and then extend the due date by a few days.

Once the ISFs are returned, the program planner will need to compare the feedback on the forms with the employee needs identified earlier in the identification phase. Often the identified needs and expressed interests by the employees will conflict. For example, suppose after the ISF has been returned, the program planner has the information in table 2.6 to work with.

As you can see, data collected during the identification phase indicates that back injuries could be a serious concern for your worksite. However, back health ranks third on collected ISFs. When the information and feedback gathered during the two phases differ, how should a program planner decide which needs and interests should receive priority? One way is to contact other area worksites; if they offer the specific program you're considering, they can tell you how well it has been received. Second, you could review the professional literature to determine what types of programs have the greatest potential for achiev-

ing a particular goal and weigh this information along with employee preferences and identified needs in a feasibility grid. For example, in considering a low-back injury prevention program, a review of the literature by the program planner revealed various studies showing that low-back injuries occur most frequently in employees with weak abdominal muscles, poor low-back flexibility, or improper lifting techniques. Thus, a back health program would have more impact if it were designed to

- appeal to at-risk employees,
- strengthen employees' abdominal muscles,
- enhance employees' low-back and hamstring flexibility, and
- motivate individuals to lift properly.

These objectives can be plugged into a feasibility grid (see table 2.7) representing the steps that must be completed in order to achieve program-specific goals. According to the sample comparison shown in table 2.7, low-back programs may have the greatest potential for making a positive impact on most of the criteria.

**Table 2.7   A Sample Feasibility Grid of Top Three Interests on Interest Survey Form (ISF)**

|  | 1st | 2nd | 3rd |
|---|---|---|---|
| Criteria | Exercise walking | Weight control | Low back |
| **PROCESS** | | | |
| 1. Appeal to employees | H | H | M |
| 2. Measurability | M | H | H |
| **IMPACT** | | | |
| 1. Strengthen abdomen | M | L | M |
| 2. Improve back flexibility | L | L | H |
| 3. Motivate proper lifting | L | L | H |
| **OUTCOME** | | | |
| 1. Reduce number of low-back injuries | L | L | H |
| 2. Reduce back-related medical care and workers' comp costs | L | L | H |

H = High, M = moderate, L = low

# Incentive Survey

## TELL US WHAT YOU WANT!

As you probably know by now, we are planning to launch new programs for you to promote your personal health and overall well-being. We hope you will be interested in these programs and want to regularly participate in the various offerings. In order to make these programs appealing to you, we're considering what types of incentives would be most popular with the majority of employees. Please take a few minutes to think about and fill in the following table. Indicate your preferences by checking the appropriate blanks. Thank you!

### Incentive Survey Table

|  | VALUE TO YOU | | |
|---|---|---|---|
| Incentive | High | Moderate | Low |
| T-shirt | | | |
| Exercise clothing | | | |
| Exercise shoes | | | |
| Wellness day off work | | | |
| Gift certificate from local store or restaurant | | | |
| Enter sweepstakes drawing | | | |
| Reduced health insurance premium | | | |
| Extended time to participate at lunchtime | | | |
| Company-paid health expense account | | | |
| Free exercise stress test | | | |
| "Well bucks" exchanged for personal items | | | |
| Other (please list): | | | |

Let's look again at the conflicting data we have received during the identification phase and from the ISF. Data collected at the identification phase clearly show that poor nutrition is a problem that should be addressed at your worksite, but good nutrition receives relatively low interest on the ISF compared to walking. What should you do? You might ask experienced WHP directors and search for available literature on the Internet to see whether nutrition programs or walking programs had better success rates. If walking has fared well as a WHP program, you might choose to launch health promotion at your worksite with a walking program because of its proven success elsewhere. As employees begin to experience the health benefits of exercise, you might then implement the idea of nutrition as a way of improving one's energy and stamina while walking. On the other hand, if you had begun health promotion at your worksite with a nutrition program, you might have met immediate resistance and thereby reduced interest in both the walking program and the WHP program overall.

You can see that properly assessing feedback from the ISF involves more than a simple quantitative evaluation. To make the best use of the ISF, you'll need to compare the results with other data and do the follow-up research necessary for viewing the ISF data in the most useful light.

## Assessing What Will Motivate Employees

Closely related to what interests employees is the issue of what will motivate them to follow up on their expressed interests. A simple way to determine the right incentives is to ask people what would motivate them to participate in a health promotion program. For example, publicize and distribute an incentive survey along with an ISF. Adapt it to your own company based on preliminary projections of your budget, program offerings, and number of employees expected to participate. The survey will provide you with a basic idea of what will attract employees, which you can combine later with the more precise information on resources that you will gather during the planning phase, discussed in chapter 3.

Assessment is a crucial phase in the framework for planning your WHP programs. Misjudgments during this phase can have a negative impact on the WHP program. Accurate assessments, however, can get WHP started off on the right track, greatly increasing the chances for long-term success.

## WHAT DO YOU THINK?

Suppose a workforce made up of 40% smokers expressed on the ISF a strong preference for walking and stress management. However, smoking appears to be one of the most prevalent risk factors in the workforce, and you think many smokers would like to quit. The human resources department has recently informed all employees that smoking will be prohibited at the worksite in 6 months. You think that smokers' stress levels will increase as the date of the no-smoking policy nears. You assume that some smokers, though not all, would participate in a walking program. What approach would you take in developing your next program to address each of these issues separately or all of them simultaneously? Would you initiate smoking cessation interventions before offering a walking program to help smokers deal with their sense of urgency? Would you offer a stress management program first as a means to help smokers kick their habit before the no-smoking policy takes effect? Or would you offer a walking program first on the premise that it will help reduce stress and, in turn, reduce the urge for smokers to smoke?

In making this important decision, what would you do to ensure that nonsmokers' preferences are not delayed because of the impending no-smoking policy? You certainly have many options to consider.

# Planning Worksite Health Promotion Programs

# Preparing Purposes and Goals

After reading this chapter you will be able to

→ Construct an appropriate mission statement and vision statement.

→ List essential parts of a goal and an objective.

→ Explain several reasons for including preliminary evaluation procedures into the planning phase.

→ Distinguish between short-term and long-term objectives.

→ List several examples of employee health indicators and organizational health indicators.

As budgets get tighter and the demands to justify spending become greater, health promotion planners must plan better than ever. In this chapter you will learn more about issues to consider during the planning phase of the framework introduced earlier (see chapter 2). Numerous surveys indicate that program planning is the most time-consuming task performed by WHP program directors. Thus, chapters 3 through 7 are devoted to various aspects of program planning. The results of the identification and assessment phases discussed in the preface should direct programming decisions. For example, as you prepare strategies to deal with the problems identified during phases 1 and 2, you should review the collected data in order to answer four questions about each problem:

1. How prevalent is the problem?
2. What are the consequences of the problem?
3. What are the causes of the problem?
4. Which workers in the company are at greatest risk?

Let's see how this process works: Imagine a company that is considering a low-back injury prevention program. Program planners in this company begin by asking an initial question: How prevalent is the problem? Data gathered during the first phase tell them that nearly one of every four employees reported a low-back pain over the past year. These numbers constitute a pervasive problem, so the planners proceed to the next question: What are the consequences of the problem? Reviewing the data, planners discover that one third of those reporting low-back pain missed more than 2 weeks of work during the previous year. What's more, they learn by exploring the third question that nearly half of the employees with back pain do not always use proper lifting methods. This information indicated to WHP planners that a program should be developed to address low-back injuries. Once this decision has been made, the fourth question is asked: Which workers in the company are at greatest risk? Again reviewing data gathered during the identification phase, planners find that the majority of those who reported low-back injury or low-back pain were men under 45 working in the shipping, foundry, or quality control departments.

So, after asking these questions, program planners understand that

- a need exists for a low-back injury program,

- a consequence of the problem is high absenteeism,
- a cause of the problem is that some workers do not know or do not use proper lifting techniques, and
- the program should be targeted mainly at men under 45 who work in one or more of three specific departments.

Armed with this information, WHP personnel can now proceed through several important steps, including (but not always in this order) the following:

1. Establishing vision and mission statements
2. Setting appropriate goals for the program
3. Making programming and resource decisions (see chapters 4, 5, and 6)
4. Funding and budgeting the program (see chapter 5)
5. Deciding whether to establish an integrated program (i.e., operate WHP within an existing department such as Human Resources) or an independent arrangement in which the program exists on its own (see chapter 7)
6. Incorporating reliable methods to evaluate the WHP program (see chapter 8)

Each of these steps in the planning process will be discussed in detail in the following sections.

## ESTABLISHING VISION AND MISSION STATEMENTS

The operating structure of an organization is a significant factor to consider in planning and implementing WHP programs. Each organization has its own unique way of planning, implementing, and sustaining its business functions to be successful. In order to understand the operating structure used by a particular organization, it would be helpful to use a Socratic approach designed around such questions as the following: What are we doing? Why are we offering this particular product or service? How are we serving the needs of our customers? With whom are we partnering to provide this service? Who is responsible for each phase of product development, marketing, and delivery? When are specific services provided to customers? And, where are we providing these

services? By answering the preceding questions, WHP program planners will have a better understanding of how their organization functions as they proceed with their own planning.

It is important for a WHP program to reflect the organization's vision and mission (see figure 3.1). One of the first tasks in planning WHP programs is to establish appropriate and clearly delineated vision and mission statements. A vision statement reflects what a WHP program aspires to achieve and its identity in the organization. With the advent of health and productivity issues gaining popularity in many worksites, WHP planners may choose a vision statement such as this one:

> WHP will be a leading contributor toward health and productivity management throughout the next decade.

Once a vision statement is established, program planners focus on an appropriate mission. The mission statement is usually more than a one-dimensional statement because it is designed to reflect a clear statement of philosophy, purpose, and goals that declares the organization's commitment for achieving the vision. For example, the following mission statement was developed by WHP planners in a large midwestern industry:

> The employee wellness program is operated to provide opportunities, services, and resources for employees, spouses, and retirees to make healthy lifestyle choices. Its purpose is to help improve health risk status and control health-related costs, with special emphasis on less-fit and at-risk participants.

The preceding statement consists of the following dimensions:

- Who we are (employee wellness program)
- What we do (provide opportunities, services, and resources)
- General population (employees, spouses, and retirees)
- Objective or prerequisite (healthy lifestyle choices)
- Employee health goal (improve health risk status)
- Organizational or corporate health goal (control health-related costs)
- Target population (less-fit and at-risk participants)

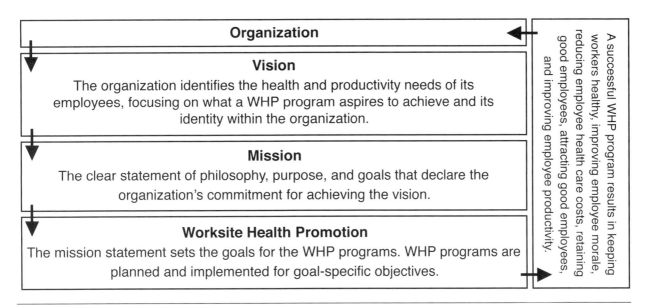

**Figure 3.1** Relationships between an organization's vision, mission, and WHP program.

Although the preceding dimensions are common in many goals, some program planners may decide to limit the scope of their goals and, thus, include only a portion of these elements.

# SETTING APPROPRIATE GOALS

For convenience, continue to use the example of a company in which low-back injury has been recognized as a pervasive problem among employees. During this first step of the planning phase, the company's WHP program planners need to establish goals that are realistic enough to attain and yet demanding enough to bring about a clear improvement in the problem area.

Both the research literature and common sense tell us that improper lifting technique is connected to back injury or pain. In our case study, almost half of the employees with back injury or pain do not always use proper lifting technique. Thus, it is reasonable to assume that reports of back injury and pain could decrease up to 50% if all employees lifted properly. If this were the case, would a program outcome of reducing low-back injuries by 50% be an appropriate goal? The answer is, probably not. Although 50% sounds like a high percentage under most circumstances, in this case the desired impact should be higher. Considering how relatively simple it should be to reduce by nearly half the number of total low-back injuries (because a single intervention—proper lifting technique—is

sufficient rather than multiple interventions), a good low-back health program should strive for closer to a 75% success rate. This would mean that 25% of all back injuries would need to be addressed through interventions other than training for proper lifting technique. Each case must be evaluated individually to establish a suitable goal for each program.

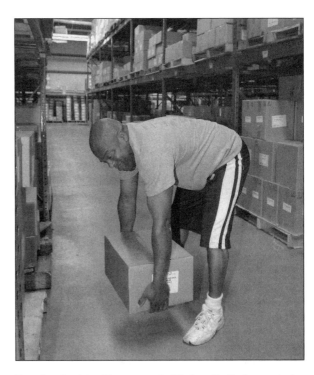

For a low-back health program in this hypothetical case study, a 75% reduction is demanding yet realistic.

# Goal Criteria

Because you are developing your evaluation goals in connection with specific programs, you must think not only about goals that are exclusively concerned with evaluation but about the general goals of the WHP programs as well. If the goals of those programs are keenly developed, it will make your evaluation goals that much easier to develop. Evaluation is greatly enhanced when the program being evaluated contains goals that are developed around the following criteria:

1. *Compatibility with stakeholders' personal health and values.* Participants, program personnel, top management, or other stakeholders value the desirable outcome.
2. *Quantifiability.* Evaluators can track and apply a statistical value (#, $, %) to the desired outcome variable.
3. *Measurability.* Evaluators can physically record changes that may occur in the outcome variable.
4. *Sufficient intervention time frame.* The intervention will be offered for a sufficient amount of time for a favorable impact to occur.
5. *Realistic achievability.* It is very likely that the intervention will favorably impact the outcome variable.

Let's take a couple of goals that are not very useful for either planning or evaluation and, by applying the five goal criteria, rewrite them until they are useful for evaluation. Suppose that your two goals are as follows:

- Improve the cardiovascular health of female employees.
- Improve employee productivity.

Now, one by one, here is how adding the elements defined in each of the criteria can transform these vaguely stated goals into valuable tools for planning both programs and evaluation:

1. Compatibility with stakeholders' personal health and values.

When you are creating your goals, you must be certain that the stakeholders will support them. Say, for example, that after you decided on your goals, you ran a survey on the 400 women in your workforce and learned that the primary health concern of 350 of them was breast cancer prevention. In that case, you would have a hard time selling your cardiovascular health program. If you had limited funds and could afford only one major program for women, you would want to change the focus of your goal. You might begin to rewrite it as, Reduce personal risk of breast cancer among female employees. Of course, you would have saved yourself some trouble had you surveyed the stakeholders in your women's health program before you decided on your goal. We will assume that you had surveyed major stakeholders already about employee productivity; thus, that goal will remain the same.

2. Quantifiability.

Although both of your goals are now compatible with the interests of your stakeholders, neither is particularly useful yet because neither contains anything that can be quantified. One way of stating this requirement for quantifiability would be to say that in order for a goal statement to be measurable, it must contain an outcome variable. An outcome variable is also known as a dependent variable and represents an observable property that varies; that is, it takes on different values, depending on the impact of the intervention (independent variable). You can improve your incomplete goals by assigning each of them a quantifiable (dependent) variable that could serve as a measurement of progress toward the general goal. Consider the following as examples:

- Reduce personal risk of breast cancer among female employees as shown by at least a 50% reduction in risk factor prevalence for breast cancer in the female workforce.
- Improve employee productivity through a reduction in on-the-job tardiness and absenteeism of at least 30%.

You can see that the second version of each goal includes a measurable factor. You can also see from the two examples that it is not possible to write measurable program goals in the absence of baseline data. You cannot, after all, tell when an improvement in anything has occurred if you do not know the original value. Thus, if no baseline exists for the area being measured, the first goal should be to establish one. For your goals, for example, you would first need to know the current breast cancer risk-factor status of the female workforce. Second, data about absenteeism are needed, such as the average tardiness rate every

6 months and average absenteeism rate every 6 months for the last 3 years. In the case of certain program evaluation goals, the baseline could be established in the first evaluation time frame.

3. Measurability.

Now that you have qualified your goals, your next step is to be sure that you have the means to measure them. Continuing with our example, you must ask yourself what resources are available for measuring breast cancer risk, on-the-job tardiness, and absenteeism. For example, will breast cancer risk be assessed using personalized health risk appraisals, self-reported feedback, clinical screening, or medical claims data? Do departmental supervisors have the proper tools to easily monitor tardiness and absenteeism?

4. Sufficient intervention time frame.

In order to know how to plan and how to evaluate, you must also include some kind of time frame in your goals. Consider these examples:

- Improve the health of female employees as shown by at least a 50% reduction in the number of women classified as high risk within 6 months.
- Improve employee productivity through a reduction in on-the-job tardiness and absenteeism of at least 30% in 4 months.

Now you have a defined target at which you can aim. Without a definite deadline to aim for, your measurement of progress is not very meaningful. Only when you know how you're doing within a time frame can you know whether you need to change your tactics to be more effective or whether it would be reasonable to set your sights higher than your original goal.

5. Realistic achievability.

It is important to establish a goal that is realistically achievable in order not to create false expectations for yourself or others. Although the goals developed so far are compatible with stakeholders' personal goals and feature both measurability and a chronological definition, you must also be sure that they are realistic. How do you do this? You can form a good idea of what is realistic in your situation by studying similar programs and learning what their results have been, as well as studying the factors that have affected their success rates. In doing so, you should look for significant differences between your situation and those of other programs studied—for example, differences in educational level, age of participants, number and types of risk factors within the target population, and cultural differences (e.g., smoking cessation efforts might not be as successful in tobacco-growing areas as in Silicon Valley). Consulting

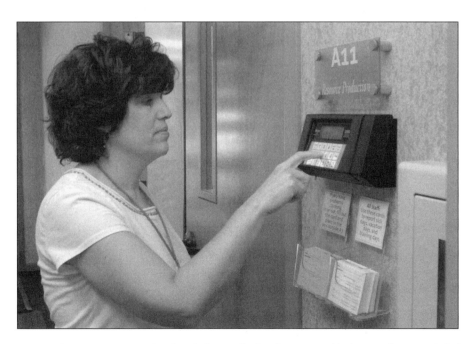

It is crucial that you secure the proper personnel and tools for monitoring the measurable factors of your goals before you proceed with your evaluation.

an expert is also a useful strategy. Once you do your homework regarding your two hypothetical goals, you discover that, in fact, they are not realistic. Based on what you have learned, then, the revisions you make to your goals are as follows:

- Improve the health of female employees as shown by at least a 25% reduction in the number of women classified as high risk within 1 year.
- Improve employee productivity through a reduction in on-the-job tardiness and absenteeism of at least 10% in 6 months.

Some evaluation experts recommend that once you establish what seem to be objective goals, you lower your sights a few percentage points to take into account differences you may have overlooked. If you have a general idea of what you'd like to accomplish in your WHP program, applying the five goal criteria to those general ideas will yield goals that are quantifiable, measurable, realistic, chronologically defined, and compatible with your stakeholders' interests. Such goals are indispensable for valid evaluation as well as for program development.

## Establishing Measurable Objectives

Once program goals have been developed, it is time to establish measurable objectives to indicate what actions must occur to attain each goal. Objectives are stepping stones, or rungs in a ladder, that enable program planners to achieve a particular goal. As an evaluator, you should be very interested in objectives because properly written objectives will facilitate and enhance the quality of the evaluation process and results.

When constructing objectives, you should do the following:

- Establish short-term objectives to use in monitoring progress in the initial phase of the intervention. For example: At the end of

## Prenatal Health Enhancement Program Objectives

- **Objective 1:** Identify population at risk. Population is female employees and dependents who experienced a pregnancy complication in the past 2 years. Evaluation planning decision: During weeks 1 through 4, contact the organization's health insurer or third-party claims administrator to obtain medical claims data on the number of all pregnancy-related complications.

- **Objective 2:** Conduct an analysis of pregnancy-related claims data from the past 2 years to identify specific types of pregnancy-related complications. Review specific complications by ICD and DRG. Evaluation planning decision: During weeks 5 through 6, develop a framework in which to record the number of each type of complication that has been incurred in the past 2 years.

- **Objective 3:** Develop an expanded prenatal screening and health education program with financial incentives. Evaluation planning decision: During weeks 7 through 8, develop a framework to track participation in the screening and education program.

- **Objective 4:** Inform all women of the new program and incentives using bulletin boards, paycheck stuffers, e-mails, and newsletters. Evaluation planning decision: During weeks 9 through 10, prepare a format to list distribution activities.

- **Objective 5:** Provide orientation sessions including a comprehensive health screening to identify women at risk of pregnancy complications; construct a format for collecting baseline data. Evaluation planning decision: During weeks 11 through 12, establish a two-group, quasi-experimental evaluation design.

- **Objective 6:** Initiate on-site programs and additional referrals to personal physicians for selected women, if necessary. Evaluation planning decision: During weeks 13 through 18, record the names and numbers of on-site participants and off-site referrals.

- **Objective 7:** Monitor health status of at-risk women at appropriate (risk-based) intervals. Provide customized interventions for each woman. Evaluation planning decision: During weeks 24 and 30, compare baseline health status levels to 6-month and 12-month levels. Analyze interval-to-interval changes to determine the intervention impact.

1 month, at least 75% of all original participants will be actively involved in personalized risk-reduction programs.

- Establish long-range objectives to determine whether initial levels of progress have been sustained. For example: At the end of 6 months, at least 50% of all participants achieving initial risk-reduction goals will have maintained or exceeded that level of success.

- Avoid the temptation to establish a long list of objectives, especially if the intervention to be evaluated is a short-term one, if evaluations have not been conducted in the past, or if an evaluation will be used as a prelude to a more formalized and thorough evaluation. Too many objectives can add unnecessary procedures that will increase the costs of conducting an evaluation.

- Include objectives that identify specific resources needed to achieve the goal. For example: Develop a health care provider network of personal physicians for all at-risk referrals.

- Specify time frames when appropriate. For example: All participants will be screened at a minimum on a quarterly basis and more frequently if they are classified in the high-risk category.

Properly written objectives are invaluable in planning the evaluation process. Suppose, for example, that the primary goal of a prenatal health enhancement program in a midsized manufacturing site (900 employees) is to increase the percentage of healthy babies at least 20% for employees and dependents within 12 months (sample objectives appear on p. 34). You can see that if all of the objectives are achieved, the goal with which they are associated will have been reached. Note that some of these objectives are not directly related to evaluation (e.g., Initiate on-site programs and additional referrals . . . ), yet the programs required by the objectives (i.e., the effectiveness of the on-site and additional referral program) will need to be evaluated. You must plan for those evaluations at this stage. The program objectives tell you what data you will need to collect, how often you will need to analyze it, and what instruments you will need to use. Each objective is followed by appropriate evaluation planning decisions you may make based on that objective.

# BUILDING EVALUATION INTO YOUR PROGRAM

Some WHP program planners make the mistake of designing an evaluation after the health promotion program is underway rather than during the planning phase. This mistake often leads to rushed evaluation procedures that yield unreliable results. Because crafting the evaluation is so important, chapter 8 is devoted to that subject. Carefully consider the information you find there; proper evaluation planning at this stage is essential for the program to achieve its potential.

Assuming appropriate goals have been set in the first place (see p. 31 for a discussion of goal setting), the best way to evaluate a program's success is to compare the program's results to the program's goals. Unfortunately, results cannot be judged until after the program has been completed. Because evaluation procedures need to be set up early, we need ways to anticipate realistic results of a program. Two good ways to gauge the potential impact of health promotion programs are to (1) talk to other WHP professionals who have implemented similar programs and (2) review the literature to see what types of programs have had a positive influence. For instance, reviewing the data in table 3.1 from published studies on WHP should help you know what to expect from a specific program and thereby help you set standards to evaluate your own program. Refer to the bibliography for examples of WHP studies on specific variables.

## Health Indicators

| Employee Health | Organizational Health |
|---|---|
| Blood pressure | Absenteeism |
| Body fat percentage | Accidents and injuries |
| Body weight | Health care usage |
| Cholesterol level | Health care costs |
| Flexibility | Productivity |
| Glucose level | Turnover |
| Coping skills (stress) | Workers' compensation costs |
| Eating habits | |
| Safety belt usage | |
| Substance abuse | |
| Tobacco use | |

**Table 3.1    Variables Directly Related to Employee Health Status and Behavior**

| Program | VARIABLES | | |
| --- | --- | --- | --- |
| | Short-term (<1 year) | Intermediate (1-2 years) | Long-term (>2 years) |
| Physical fitness | Health status | Absenteeism | Health care costs |
| Nutrition and weight control | Health status<br>Productivity<br>Blood pressure | Health care usage | Health care costs |
| Back health | Back injuries<br>Productivity | Health care usage | Health care costs |
| Prenatal health | Health status<br>Health insurance<br>Productivity | Absenteeism<br>Health care usage<br>Turnover | Health care costs |
| Smoking control | Health status<br>Health insurance<br>Property insurance | Absenteeism<br>Health care usage | Health care costs |
| AIDS education and HIV disease prevention | Absenteeism<br>Health status<br>Productivity | Health care usage | Health care costs |
| Medical self-care and health care consumerism | Self-care confidence | Health care usage | Health care costs |
| Occupational injury | Health care usage<br>Productivity<br>Work satisfaction | Turnover | Accident costs |
| Employee assistance program (EAP) and quality of work life (QWL) | Health status<br>Mental health<br>Work satisfaction | Absenteeism<br>Accidents<br>Health care usage<br>Productivity<br>Work satisfaction<br>EAP usage | Health care costs |
| Stress management | Coping skills<br>Health status | Health care usage | Health care costs |

Variables directly related to employee health status and behavior are called employee health indicators. Variables closely related to an organization's health and productivity are called organizational health indicators. A sampling of each category can be seen on page 35.

Some indicators may be defined and measured according to a specific company's operations, philosophy, and record-keeping practices. Take absenteeism, for example. Many companies classify absences as either scheduled or unscheduled. Some typical examples of both classifications are listed next.

Because WHP programs have no impact on factors that prompt scheduled factors, program goals and evaluation procedures should focus on

## Absence Classifications

| Controllable (Unscheduled) | Uncontrollable (Scheduled) |
| --- | --- |
| Poor health or illness | Jury duty or military duty |
| Falsely calling in "sick" | |
| Work-related disability | Maternity or paternity leave |
| Faking an injury | Attending a funeral |
| | Inclement weather |

factors that prompt unscheduled absences. See chapter 8 for a complete discussion of evaluation procedures.

## WHAT WOULD YOU DO?

Senior management recently gave all midlevel managers, including your boss, a mandate to demonstrate that every employee service program is closely aligned to the organization's vision and mission statement. Its current vision is to become the world's leading supplier of computers to business and industry. Its mission is to provide a culture for workers to be the most productive and cost-efficient workers in the industry. Although the company's mission is void of any direct reference to employee health, your boss asks you to prepare a WHP vision and mission focused on productivity. Yet, you feel a person's health and productivity are strongly related. Thus, you would like to incorporate something about health and productivity in either your vision or mission statement. You realize the need to diplomatically convince your boss to see your side. How would you consider sharing any published research as evidence to justify your position? Would you research what other companies in the industry have done in this area?

# Selecting Healthy Lifestyle Programs

**4**

After reading this chapter you will be able to

→ Cite several major factors to consider in selecting specific types of WHP programs.

→ Distinguish between the traditional fitness center–based approach and the evolving holistic life center–based approach.

→ List several ways to create healthier eating options at a worksite.

→ Describe a sample step-by-step process for establishing a worksite no-smoking policy.

**E**ach worksite has unique needs that require particular WHP programs and resources. This portion of chapter 4 presents an overview of various programs, including physical fitness, back health, weight control, prenatal health, smoking cessation, HIV/AIDS education, medical self-care, financial wellness, budgeting, and programming philosophy.

## PHYSICAL FITNESS

One of the most pressing challenges facing WHP program directors today is how to motivate employees to exercise on a regular basis. The Surgeon General's Report on Physical Activity and Health advises people to do at least 30 minutes a day of moderate exercise (e.g., walking at 3 or 4 miles per hour). Currently, fewer than one of every five American adults meet this standard. In 2005, the Department of Health and Human Services (DHHS) and the United States Department of Agriculture (USDA) jointly released the Dietary Guidelines for Americans 2005, which recommends at least 30 minutes of moderate-

intensity physical activity (not counting usual activity) on most days of the week. However, it states that for most people, greater health benefits can be obtained by engaging in activity that is more intense or for a longer duration. The recommendations encourage not only cardiovascular conditioning but also stretching for flexibility and resistance exercises or calisthenics for muscle strength and endurance. For those wanting to prevent weight gain, DHHS recommends 60 minutes of moderate to vigorous exercise on most days of the week. For those wishing to drop pounds, 60 to 90 minutes of daily, moderate-intensity exercise is advised. (Dietary Guidelines for Americans, 2005)

For the first time in the history of the world, the percentage of inactive adults exceeds the percentage of active adults, and this startling statistic extends to the workplace. In hopes of motivating employees to exercise, many employers provide **physical fitness programs** (PFPs) stemming from the following:

- Growing evidence showing regular exercise can reduce the risk of heart disease, cancer, stroke (the leading causes of death), and many other conditions

- Increasing evidence of a direct relationship between physical activity and on-the-job productivity
- Growing frustration of paying billions of dollars to treat many illnesses and disorders that can be prevented by a physically active lifestyle
- Efforts to regain a competitive edge by improving employee health
- Growing appeal of fitness center or health club benefits by employees and job applicants

If you are interested in calculating the economic cost of physical inactivity in your community or organization, check out the physical inactivity cost calculator, sponsored by Active Living Leadership and the Robert Wood Johnson Foundation. It can be accessed at: www.activelivingleadership.org.

More WHP programs are shifting from a predominant focus on a fitness center–based PFP to a holistic (total wellness oriented) life center approach. By doing so, worksites are trying to soften the emphasis on physical health, cardiovascular conditioning, and strength training. Consequently, this approach may involve a resource or support center designed to encourage employees to explore a broad range of life issues (relationships, financial wellness, rest and play, aging, mind–body healing, spirituality, and so on). Essentially, PFPs of all shapes and sizes can be integrated into a person's lifestyle and directly contribute to the quality of their aging process, financial health, recreational pursuits, spiritual connections, and healing. Simultaneously, this holistic approach to exercise programming creates experiences for individuals to explore the mind–body–spirit connection through movement rather than exercising solely to reshape the body, lose weight, or compensate for overeating.

While some of today's more publicized PFPs operate in modern, state-of-the-art, multi-million-dollar fitness centers, most worksites do not have the need, much less the financial resources, for constructing such facilities. Many of these sites instead provide small, on-site fitness centers or subsidize employee memberships to local health clubs. Some worksites combine various strategies within their health management framework, sometimes using a cafeteria plan to better meet the diverse needs of their employees.

# Exercise Precautions

Although heart attacks during exercise are rare, most health clubs and worksite fitness centers take certain precautionary measures to handle such possibilities. The most common safeguards involve having staff members trained in and capable of administering cardiopulmonary resuscitation (CPR) as well as having an in-house communication system to notify emergency medical personnel immediately in the event of a life-threatening event. In addition, the topic of automated early defibrillators (AEDs) is generating much attention as more states consider passing laws for exercise facilities. Although the bulk of the early mandates was directed primarily at commercial health clubs, some industry insiders feel that WHP programs will follow. And with a noted study published in the *Journal of the American Medical Association* showing that CPR is often performed inadequately by even trained medical professionals, pressure to make AEDs more readily available will continue to mount in all exercise facilities (Brown and Kellerman, 2000). Adding to the pressure being felt by some

## AED Risk Management

According to the Early Defibrillator Law and Policy Center (EDLPC), as AEDs become more common, a higher risk exists for organizations that fail to purchase and properly use these devices. To reduce this risk, exercise facilities need to develop a cardiac arrest survival system, not just buy an AED. The program must do all of the following:

- Comply with all current and future applicable local, state, and federal legal and regulatory requirements
- Meet life-saving response-time goals
- Be designed for the unique characteristics of each program site
- Properly configure the people, systems, methods, equipment, and actions required to save lives
- Create an environment that encourages life-saving action
- Properly balance system costs, benefits, and risks
- Be thoughtful, defensible, and well documented

legislators—and eventually commercial and corporate fitness directors—is increasing activity on the judicial side of the equation. So far, several states have passed legislation mandating the placement of AEDs in health clubs. Nonetheless, it should be noted that at the time of this book's publishing, the standards of neither the American Heart Association (AHA), the American College of Sports Medicine (ACSM), nor the International Health, Racquet and Sportsclub Association (IHRSA) require the use of AEDs.

# Equipment and Facility Considerations

Designing and equipping a healthy worksite requires considerable planning and coordination between the company and outside vendors. Considering today's options, a company needs to look closely at its budget and the marketplace, review product literature, and consult with other worksite personnel. Some of your early decisions about facility planning and equipment purchasing could make or break your program, so research as much as you can before making a choice.

Purchasing equipment may take the most planning and budgeting expertise. Equipment costs vary widely, depending on brand name, durability, computerized features, and shipping expense. In general, stationary bikes cost from $300 to $3,000; multistation weight systems go for $1,000 and up; climbing machines from $1,000 to $4,000; rowers from $300 to $1,500; and treadmills from $400 to $5,000. With such a huge range in quality and price of equipment, it is foolish not to shop around. Here are some tips for purchasing equipment:

- Purchase equipment designed for institutional use.
- To cut shipping costs, buy from a local firm or manufacturer whenever possible.
- To save up to 50% off the retail price, buy carpet directly from the manufacturing mill.
- Ask distributors if they provide free equipment instruction.
- Closely compare maintenance requirements of mechanized equipment and computerized equipment.
- Check a firm's stock inventory, credit plan, warranty, service contract, and whether or not the manufacturer has product liability insurance.
- Ask vendors for the names of other companies who have purchased their equipment, and solicit opinions before buying.
- Invite sales representatives to visit your worksite to discuss your particular needs.

# Maintaining Fitness Equipment

The durability of a fitness facility and equipment is best preserved by maintaining a temperature near 70 °F (~21 °C) and humidity level lower than 50%. Ask exercisers to put a towel over computer control panels to protect them from perspiration. Place electronic equipment in locations with adequate ventilation to reduce heat overload. Monitor equipment use to ensure that it is being used properly. Misuse is probably the biggest contributor to broken or malfunctioning equipment, so provide mandatory orientation sessions for all users.

The furnishings of the facility should not only be practical but also contribute positively to the exercise environment. Fans help a facility's air conditioner circulate air more efficiently; large ceiling fans are more attractive than floor models. Mirrors should be shatterproof, especially in the weight room.

The lighting of the facility should be bright enough for safety, yet as pleasant and energy-efficient as possible. When properly positioned, windows provide natural, inexpensive lighting. Consider energy-efficient bulbs, which are more expensive up front, but more cost-efficient in the long run because they use less energy and last longer. Windows should be ideally positioned to absorb sunlight for solar heat during winter months without causing glare. Select lighting panels that provide dim lighting during off-peak hours to cut energy consumption. Mercury-vapor fluorescent bulbs work well for racquetball and basketball. Avoid surface-mounted fluorescent lights because they cause glare. If you have locker rooms, recessed fluorescent lighting provides a nice ambience.

Efficient ventilation in the shower room is essential for providing comfort, containing heating and cooling costs, and maintaining the overall health of the facility. A heating, ventilation, and air conditioning (HVAC) system that ventilates at least 40 cubic feet per minute is necessary to minimize excessive heat and moisture in showers and locker rooms.

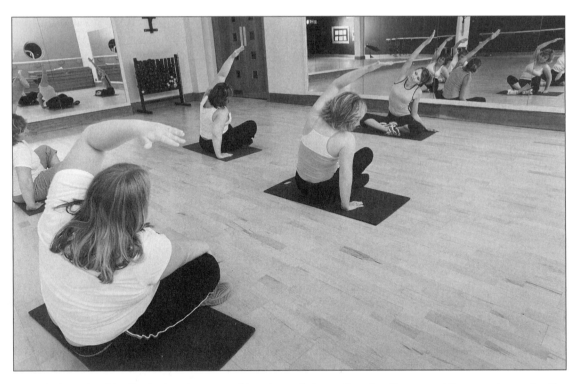

Mirrors give the best visual feedback when they are positioned on only two walls rather than around the room. Large standing plants such as parlor palms positioned in corners provide a natural look and help clean the air.

If your company can afford lockers, full-size lockers are desirable to hang dresses and suits, whereas stacked lockers are adequate for leisure clothing. A good locker has vents for air circulation, is easy to clean, is purchased from a reputable manufacturer, includes a service contract, and can be purchased at a discount when bought in bulk.

Many experts recommend surfacing your facility with a wood spring-coil floor or a polyurethane mixed-foam floor with padding or carpeting treated with stain repellant to prevent mildew. Rubber is also popular; although it is slightly more expensive than carpet or wood, it lasts longer. The cost per square foot for synthetic foam generally runs from $4.50 to $10, good carpeting from $3.50 to $5, wood from $8 to $15, and rubber from $9 to $17. If your site will include a basketball court, the best surface is polyurethane-finished wood (maple, beech, or birch), pure polyurethane, or polyurethane with acrylic resin. Prices for these surfaces run from $10 to $15 per square foot. For a racquetball court, choose a wood surface of maple, beech, or birch, costing from $10 to $15 per square foot. For high-traffic surfaces, the best choice is a synthetic-fiber carpeting of nylon or olefin, which runs from $5 to $10 per square foot. To avoid fraying, unraveling, and packing down,

select a cut-pile version with a low pile height and tight gauge construction. Choose action backing over jute backing to avoid moisture buildup and mildew. When choosing exercising flooring, consider how well a particular surface compares to established performance standards. One of the most common international protocols that many flooring vendors use is the DIN standard 18032, Part 2. DIN is a nongovernmental organization established to promote the development of standardization and related activities in Europe with the goal of facilitating the international exchange of goods and services. The particular standards are shown in table 4.1.

In the weight room, high-quality wood is a good surface. Rubber mats (with trip-free beveled edging) should be placed under each piece of equipment and in the free-weight areas to absorb sound and cushion dropped weights.

In the locker room area (if your company can afford this amenity), carpeting provides comfort, economy, safety, and easy maintenance. The carpet should have antifungus protection and be regularly wet-vacuumed and treated with stain repellant. The color or pattern should minimize the sight of visible stains. In the shower and drying area of the locker room, the best shower surface is slightly abrasive, nonslip tile. Tiles

**Table 4.1　International Standards on Key Performance Measures for Exercise Floors.**

| Floor test | DIN standard |
|---|---|
| Shock absorption | Minimum: 53% |
| Resilience | Minimum: 2.3 mm |
| Surface friction | Minimum: 0.5<br>Maximum: 0.7 |
| Impact isolation | W 500<br>Maximum: 15% |
| Surface stability | Minimum: 1,500 N |

set in mortar are less likely to fall out than tiles glued to waterproof gypsum board. Soft brown is a popular color and doesn't show stains as much as white. Shower walls should be tiled and sealed with epoxy. Epoxy sealant is relatively inexpensive and can be steam cleaned.

If you're lucky enough to afford a facility with an indoor track, choose synthetic surfaces such as rubber or a vinyl laminated to a sponge-rubber cushion. Latex, full-poured urethane, and vented urethane also work well. Corners should be banked slightly to minimize stress on the lower leg. (Remind users to alternate direction on a daily basis to reduce stress on one side of the body.)

If your company plans an outdoor fitness trail, your best selections for surface materials are decomposed granite, limestone quarry particulates, crushed coral, and wood chips. When constructing a trail, cut a 3.5-inch deep trough with a landscaping tractor. The dirt wells up on the sides of the trough, creating a natural border that holds the surface material in place. Fill the trough with 2 inches of compacted gravel, and top it with a surface material to make the trail level with the ground. Locate the trail away from office buildings so that workers are not distracted by people passing by. For one-way traffic only, a 4-foot path is adequate. You'll need a 7-foot path or bigger for two-way traffic. Provide distance markers and perhaps a bench or par course along the trail. Finally, develop procedures to enhance personal safety for all trail users. For example, require all individual users to sign their name in addition to their departing and expected return times in a highly visible location for staff members to regularly monitor. A video surveillance system may also be appropriate in specific settings.

# NUTRITION AND WEIGHT CONTROL

Worldwide, over one half of all workers are overweight or obese, and about two thirds of all workers eat unhealthy diets. High-fat diet is a major risk factor for health problems associated with many health care claims (circulatory, digestive, cancer, and metabolic), and obese individuals have significantly longer hospital stays and incur higher health care costs than their coworkers. Given these facts, it's little wonder that nutrition and weight control are prime target areas for WHP.

Developing countries are adopting lifestyles that have existed in the United States and western Europe for decades, such as working at sedentary jobs, driving cars, eating poorly, and generally being physically inactive. These lifestyles are leading to a global epidemic of obesity. An interesting case study is the Arabian Gulf countries, which, overall, don't have aging problems because they have fairly young populations. Yet, their newly acquired lifestyles have dramatically changed their illness and disease patterns. For example, rates of obesity and diabetes in the United Arab Emirates (UAE), Saudi Arabia, Kuwait, and Qatar are increasing dramatically. In particular, the prevalence of diabetes in the UAE is estimated to be at least 15%, about twice the rate in North America and Europe. Although these nations are wealthy and building high-tech medical clinics, no amount of money or technology in the world can reverse the debilitating effects of these lifestyle trends. Essentially, only lifestyle changes can improve this situation.

A review of 316 studies that evaluated various types of WHP programs over the past two decades found positive results for weight control programs; borderline positive results for nutrition, exercise, and cholesterol-reduction programs; and weak results for health risk appraisals. One of the common denominators found in successful weight control and nutrition programs was a healthy and supportive worksite culture. By incorporating this theme, WHP personnel can promote healthier eating and better weight control for employees in several ways:

- Distribute and publicize nutritional educational materials in the cafeteria and near canteens, vending machines, or break areas.
- Offer heart-healthy entrées, a salad bar, and other healthy options.

- Affix "healthy choice" labels to foods that are low in fat, calories, sugar, salt, and cholesterol.
- Offer a weekly menu of nutritious bag lunches that employees can prepare.
- Offer discounted prices on heart-healthy entrées in the cafeteria.
- Ease out the junk food from vending machines and replace it with natural fruits, unsweetened fruit juices, low-fat dairy products, and other nutritious foods. (Do not try to get rid of all junk food at once!)
- Place weight scales and body mass index (BMI) charts in company restrooms for employees to regularly monitor their weight.
- Provide free body fat measurements at quarterly intervals. Skinfold calipers are relatively inexpensive and relatively accurate when used appropriately.

Consider your options and goals before committing to purchase program resources. For example, a multifaceted program of screenings, exercise sessions, competitions, and follow-up counseling sessions may be a cost-effective approach to impact high-risk employees with multiple health problems. Weight control programs may consist of small group sessions, large group lectures, self-management tips, or weight loss competitions. Yet, in reality, most weight control programs produce little, if any, long-term success because they don't help participants regain a normal relationship with food by addressing chronic dieting, body dissatisfaction, and cultural weight prejudice.

A good resource to use in nutrition education and weight control programs is the Dietary Guidelines for Americans (www.healthierus. gov/dietaryguidelines/), which provides science-based advice to promote health and to reduce risk for chronic diseases through diet and physical inactivity. The Dietary Guidelines are published jointly every 5 years by the Department of Health and Human Services (DHHS) and the United States Department of Agriculture (USDA). The latest version of the Dietary Guidelines was released in January 2005.

Timing is an important consideration to promote healthy eating. For example, lunchtime is a good opportunity to offer lunch-and-learn seminars on such issues as cholesterol reduction, hypertension control, and diabetes control. March is National Nutrition Month, an excellent time to introduce new programs for workers shaping up

## Impact of Worksite Programs—Weight Control

What impact can a weight-reduction and nutrition education program have on employees? Here are some examples:

- **L.L. Bean Company:** 70% of the 77 Heart Club members had 14% lower cholesterol levels within 8 months, which cut their heart disease risk by 28%.
- **Campbell Soup Company:** Two hundred thirty-three employee participants in Campbell's STRIP (Spare Tire Reduction Incentive Program) lost 3,078 pounds within 3 months.
- **Dow Chemical:** The company's Walk-A-Weigh program was offered in 23 countries and 9 languages and had over 5,000 participants. It featured a nautical theme on the importance of physical activity and weight management. Over two thirds of participants reporting their results cumulatively lost 9,460 pounds.
- **DuPont:** DuPont's weight loss program produced an average weight loss of 5.5 pounds per participant; 85% of them maintained the loss at least 3 months.
- **Lockheed Missile and Space Company:** Employees lost a total of 14,378 pounds in the company's 3-month "Take It Off" program, at a cost of only $.94 per lost pound.
- **Lycoming County, Pennsylvania, businesses:** Three independent weight loss competitions between various industries and banks produced an average weight loss of 12 pounds per participant.
- **Scherer Brothers Lumber:** This company of 150 employees made its worksite healthier by removing candy machines and adding fruit dispensers, replacing caffeinated coffee with decaf, and offering healthy snacks free of charge. The new changes were welcomed by most workers as evidenced by sales receipts and healthy snack consumption.

for the summer. Several resources for consideration can be found on the Web site of the American Dietetic Association (www.eatright.org)

# BACK HEALTH

Back injury is one of the most common on-the-job injuries at the worksite and the primary cause of absenteeism in many companies. Nearly 2% of the U.S. workforce files a low-back injury claim each year; most are classified as a minor low-back muscle strain, which costs employers about $500 per injury in medical care and lost productivity costs. However, more serious back injuries such as a bulging disk, intervertebral disk disorder, or fractured vertebrae can cost around $30,000 per case. These types of back and spinal injuries comprise up to 50% of all workers' compensation claims and, thus, can lead to long-term disability in some cases.

By establishing on-site programs, many companies are reducing the incidence and cost of low-back injuries. Research indicates that the most successful low-back programs include these three major components:

- Prevention and health promotion
- Intervention and treatment for injured employees
- Rehabilitation and a return-to-work protocol

Treatment and rehabilitation of injured workers is usually provided by occupational health nurses, physical therapists, massage therapists, and other allied health care personnel, but WHP professionals often play a major role in the promotion of back health.

Perhaps the most effective incentive to promote healthy backs at the worksite is constant support from management, supervisors, and coworkers. Here are some ideas for promoting healthy back practices at your worksite:

- *Awareness and knowledge.* Make employees aware of the risk of back and spinal injuries by providing company- and industry-specific data, teaching the structure and function of the spine and lower back, and providing instructions on how to identify high-risk tasks by showing slides or videotapes of employees performing work functions. You can reinforce important learning and behavioral concepts with poster campaigns, paycheck stuffers, monthly safety meetings, and other highly visible methods. Display posters of easy stretching routines at key locations, and use the company newsletter and e-mail communications to illustrate spinal anatomy and tips on proper body mechanics for lifting, pulling, and pushing.

- *Practice.* A trained leader teaches employees proper body mechanics for lifting, bending, carrying, pushing, pulling, and reaching; employees practice prework stretching and strengthening

## Impact of Worksite Programs—Back-Injury Prevention

What impact can on-site back-injury prevention programs have on employees? Here are a few examples of the payoff in some organizations:

- **Biltrite Corporation (Chelsea, MA):** Within 1 year of operation, the company's back program produced a 90% drop ($150,000 savings) in workers' compensation back claims.

- **Capital Wire and Cable (Plano, TX):** The company saved more than $83,000 within 20 months of instituting a new low-back health program.

- **Coca-Cola Bottling Company (Atlanta, GA):** Plant employees perform a 10-minute prework routine to prepare for the rigors of loading and unloading beverage trucks. Accidents have dropped 83% and produced

annual savings of over $250 per employee in lost time and replacement costs.

- **Lockheed Missile and Space Company (Sunnyvale, CA):** The company reported a 67.5% drop in low-back injury costs within 14 months of implementing its back-health program.

- **Pepsi Bottling Group (Riviera Beach, FL, and Pompano Beach, FL):** The company reported that low-back injuries dropped from 146 to 13 within 2 years of a mandatory prework stretching program.

- **Swedish factory workers:** One weekly 30-minute session of group calisthenics combined with a 10-minute talk on low-back health resulted in fewer low-back injuries as well as a decline in sick leave absences.

routines on a daily basis with their immediate supervisor and coworkers.

• *Implementation and follow-up.* All employees are trained to lead their coworkers in daily prework stretching and strengthening exercises. Offering these sessions on company time is a good measure to show employees that their employer is investing in their health while building a cohesive, team-oriented workforce. Consider using extrinsic incentives to encourage employee participation in prework stretching and warm-up routines. For example, injury-free employees at regular intervals (3, 6, 9, and 12 months) can enter a sweepstakes to win one or more prizes presented at designated company functions or at the end of the year or receive semi-annual financial bonuses from any back-injury prevention savings.

# PRENATAL HEALTH

A full-term delivery without complications costs about $3,500 in the United States. However, a pregnancy with complications can cost an employer over $100,000. Some of this expense can be passed on to employees through higher insurance premiums, deductibles, and co-payments.

Statistics show the percentage of unhealthy infants born in most countries is an international challenge, even in the largest industrialized nations. For example, China's infant death rate is over 24 per 1,000 live births; the United States' rate is about one third this rate while Canada's 4.75, Australia's 4.69, and Japan's 3.26 rates reflect the best in the world. (In the United States, 1 of every 8 babies is born prematurely and 1 of every 14 American babies is born with a low birth weight; medical care costs for premature infants is over $5 billion a year. The hospital bill for one premature infant can be as high as $500,000, whereas a baby born with breathing or feeding problems may require more than $60,000 of health care services in a single month. Given these numbers and their impact on increasing insurance premiums, it only makes sense that employers develop aggressive programs on prenatal care as a part of their WHP efforts.

A typical prenatal health education program consists of the following components:

• *Prepregnancy counseling.* Employees interested in learning about their genetic predisposition are encouraged to meet with an occupational health nurse to discuss various issues such as influence of age, family history, pregnancy history, lifestyle, health status, and.

• *Identification.* Employees who believe they are pregnant are asked to visit the company's on-site nurse or personal physician for a pregnancy (urine) test.

• *Referral.* If an employee is pregnant, she is informed of the company's health care (maternity) benefits and referred to her personal physician; to qualify for maternity health care benefits, pregnant employees and dependents are required to attend on-site prenatal health education classes.

• *Education classes.* In conjunction with regular visits to their personal physicians (or on-site physician), pregnant women participate in the

## Financial Impact of Pregnancy Complications

To better understand the financial impact of pregnancy-related complications on some employers, consider what happened at two Oster-Sunbeam (O-S) worksites. In 1 year, four severely ill babies were born to employees at one O-S worksite; medical care costs for the four infants totaled $500,000. The next year, at the other O-S worksite, three more babies were born prematurely; one infant's lengthy hospitalization exhausted the company's major medical insurance allocation and resulted in the termination of coverage. Soon after, the company established a prenatal program that has slashed the average cost per birth by 90%. Within a year of establishing the new prenatal health education program, the cost per maternity case at the Coushatta, Louisiana, plant dropped from $27,242 to $2,893; the average cost per case at the Holly Springs, Mississippi, plant dropped from $3,500 to $2,872. Moreover, only one premature birth has occurred at either plant since the start of the program. Obviously, not all complications are preventable. However, the preceding case study at O-S as well as many similar cases reflect the influence that quality on-site prenatal health promotion interventions can have on many potentially avoidable complications (Business and Health, 1991).

## The Southern Regional Corporate Coalition to Improve Maternal and Child Health

One of the most ambitious worksite-based prenatal health promotion initiatives is the Southern Regional Corporate Coalition to Improve Maternal and Child Health. Established in 1986 by the Southern Governors' Association's Project on Infant Mortality, the Coalition consists of 29 employers from 17 southern states. Coalition studies suggest that employers will have a healthier and more productive workforce as well as cut their own expenses if they do the following:

1. Include a maternal and infant health benefit in their insurance packages with incentives to encourage families to use preventive services such as prenatal care for pregnant women.

2. Review their maternity leave policies and grant such leave for pregnant women without compromising a successful return to work.

3. Engage in public and private partnerships to develop health care public policy to encourage good maternal health.

4. Provide educational programs for employees and their families on preventive health care for mothers and children

Items 1 through 3 here generally are the concern of human resources and benefits managers. But WHP personnel are often responsible for writing and implementing educational programs on prenatal, infant, maternal, and child health.

company's prenatal health education program taught by a certified professional. One-hour programs are offered every 2 weeks on company time, and they typically include two phases:

1. *Information phase:* prenatal care, nutrition, substance use and abuse, discomforts of pregnancy, fetal development, signs and symptoms of labor and birthing, and recommendations of postnatal home care.

2. *Clinical phase:* one-on-one screenings and discussions to assess each woman's blood pressure, weight, water retention level, and urine test results.

In between classes, informal sessions are held for women who are in the later stages of pregnancy or are considered high risk because of excess weight, hypertension, or a history of difficult childbirth.

The Colorado Department of Health Affairs estimates that at least $9 could be saved for every dollar spent on prenatal care. If long-term costs were included, the savings could be as much as $11 for every dollar spent. Numerous companies including Cigna, First Chicago Bank, and O-S have reported impressive cost savings from their prenatal health education programs.

A high participation level of pregnant employees (especially those at risk) is vital to the overall success of any prenatal health education program. Although many companies have mandatory par-

ticipation policies (to qualify for 100% employer-paid maternity benefits), employees tend to take a more genuine interest in prenatal programs that include personal incentives. Some of the more successful incentives include the following:

• Offering programs on company time

• Waiving the first year health insurance deductible and co-payment if the expectant mother attends all scheduled prenatal classes

• Offering monetary rewards (e.g., $100) for attending all scheduled prenatal classes and screening sessions

• Paying a higher percentage (e.g., 100% versus 80%) of the health care bill for participating mothers.

The actual effectiveness of specific incentives will vary from worksite to worksite, so incentives should be tailored around employees' needs and interests, the worksite culture, and an employer's financial situation. Management can make a significant impact on mothers and babies by taking the following actions:

• Sponsor a meeting of management and supervisors to announce company support of a prenatal health promotion program (i.e., March of Dimes' New Beginnings). Explain the purpose, clarify the benefits to the company and the employees, and gain commitment for your program.

- Involve employee representatives and supervisors in your efforts. Solicit their help to recruit employees, promote the program, and offer ideas on how to get the message out.
- Send a personalized letter of invitation to every employee announcing your company's support.
- Appoint one or more employees or volunteers to be representatives for healthy mothers and healthy babies programs. Have special buttons, name tags, or T-shirts made for these representatives. Responsibilities may include giving presentations to employee groups and meetings, placing articles or announcements in company newsletters, changing bulletin boards and posters, and creating novel ways to promote the programs. Provide recognition and support for these representatives and rotate their appointments occasionally to prevent burnout and to give others a chance to contribute.
- Publicize your maternity-related health policies and benefits, and emphasize the importance of early prenatal care.
- Link your company name and logo with the prenatal program. For example: "ABC Company and New Beginnings: Working Together for Healthy Moms and Healthy Babies."

Companies are discovering that investing in prenatal and maternal health programs pays off. Each high-risk pregnancy that is avoided saves tens, if not hundreds, of thousands of dollars for employers and society, and it translates into healthier families, communities, and workforces in the future.

# SMOKING CONTROL

One of the most visible examples of business' commitment to employees' health is reflected in the growth of smoking control policies at many worksites. Nearly three fourths of all medium and large worksites throughout North America have smoking control policies, and most of these organizations also offer smoking cessation programs. In addition, more European worksites became smoke-free after Italy, Malta, and Ireland established indoor clean air policies in 2005.

Many factors are responsible for business' growing push for smoke-free worksites. First, federal agencies are addressing the issue in various ways. The 2004 U.S. Surgeon General's Report attributes an estimated 420,000 deaths each year to cigarette smoking, making it one of the nation's leading causes of preventable death; in 1986, the General Services Administration (GSA) significantly restricted smoking in 6,800 federal office buildings; and in 1990, the Environmental Protection Agency (EPA) officially classified secondhand smoke as a significant indoor pollutant and a class A carcinogen. Second, antidrug campaigns are spreading into worksites and targeting illegal drugs as well as legal drugs such as cigarettes (nicotine). Third, more nonsmokers are requesting their employers to establish smoke-free working environments. Fourth, more business owners are becoming aware of the economic costs of smoking employees; smokers are absent an average of 2 to 5 days more per year than nonsmokers and incur approximately 15%

## Smoking Control Policy Benefits

Potential benefits to employers who establish smoking control policies include, but are not limited to the following:

- Lower health, life, and fire insurance and workers' compensation premium costs
- Fewer health care claims and costs from smoking-related conditions (see table 4.2)
- Less absenteeism from smoking-related illnesses
- Less property and equipment damage and lower maintenance costs
- Fewer accidents and reduced fire risk
- Greater productivity (avoidance of "down time" used for smoking breaks)
- Fewer premature disabilities and deaths from cigarette smoking

Actual benefits depend largely on factors such as the extent of smoking control measures; the amount of smoking and physiological damage to the heart, lungs, and blood vessels before such measures are implemented; the percentage of employees who smoke off-site; the general health of workers; and coexposure to other occupational hazards such as asbestos, coal dust, and so on.

**Table 4.2  Economic Cost of Cigarette Smoking in 1976 and 2006**

| Cost category | 1976 | 2006 |
| --- | --- | --- |
| Lost production | $19.13 billion | $62.07 billion |
| Direct health care | $8.22 billion | $71.99 billion |
| Total | $27.36 billion | $134.06 billion |

1976 costs provided by the New England Journal of Medicine (Vol. 11, No. 298, 1978). Year 2006 cost estimates provided by the author using the following rates of inflation: lost production based on 4% annual inflation; direct health care costs based on 7.5% annual medical care inflation.

higher health care costs than nonsmokers. Fifth, strong evidence exists that smoking employees incur greater medical care and lost productivity costs than nonsmoking workers. Finally, a growing body of statutory, regulatory, and judicial developments exist that

- grant employees the right to sue employers if smoking is permitted in a workplace;
- stipulate that employers can be held partially accountable for employee pain, discomfort, and illness caused by tobacco smoke in the workplace; and
- rule that no legal grounds exist for claims that smoking at work is a "constitutional right."

Additional factors influencing worksite smoking control efforts include ensuring the purity of manufactured products, preventing property and equipment damage, and enhancing a company's corporate image to shareholders and the public.

## Program and Policy Planning

Early employer initiatives to reduce smoking prevalence focused on policies and programs delivered at the worksite. Overall, policy-level changes are effective in reducing the prevalence of worksite smoking at least 10% more than worksites without such policies.

Worksite-based smoking cessation programs include self-help manuals, physician advice, health education, cessation groups, and competitions. Although effective, these programs have been plagued by low participation rates. Incentives have produced some effectiveness in increasing participation rates, but this does not necessarily translate to improved cessation rates.

Some tools for quitting smoking and some common brands and prices are as follows:

*Nicotine Replacement Therapies*

- Gum: Nicorette—over the counter; $4.50 for 10 pieces
- Inhaler: Plastic cylinder containing a cartridge that delivers nicotine when you puff on it; $45 per package (42 cartridges)
- Nasal spray: Nicotrol NS—prescription required; $5 per day for average use (13 doses) or $15 per day for maximum usage (40 doses)
- Patch: Nicoderm—both over the counter and prescription; $4 per day

*Non-Nicotine Prescription Drugs*

- Bupropion—marketed under the brand name Zyban, also sold as the antidepressant Wellbutrin, $2 per day; generic, $1.17 per day

*Counseling*

- Quit lines: state or federal (1-800-QUIT-NOW) hotline; free
- Private telephone-based counseling: Average $200 to $300 for four to six intensive phone conversations
- Group counseling in smoking cessation: Offered through public health departments, nonprofit groups such as the American Cancer Society, and commercial groups such as SmokEnders and SmokeStoppers; session prices range from $50 to $350

When planning a smoking control policy, a program director should properly structure and communicate the strategy for establishing smoke-free initiatives at the worksite. For example, more worksites are integrating their smoke-free efforts within clean air policy proposals and the theme of protecting the health of employees. This minimizes the potential for heated debates, personal conflicts, and friction between smoking employees and management.

So-called half-and-half policies (banning smoking at workstations only) are essentially counterproductive because they force smokers to leave their work areas to smoke, resulting in lost productivity. In contrast, a total clean air worksite policy can eliminate such violations and also help smokers who are trying to quit. Removing

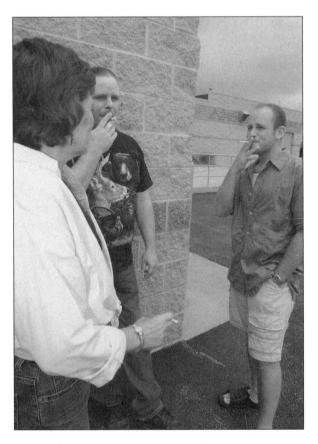

An excellent time to implement smoking cessation activities and policy changes is during the Great American Smokeout sponsored by the American Cancer Society each November or the Canadian Cancer Society's National Non-Smoking Week in January.

all cigarette vending machines from the worksite and providing smoking cessation programs with financial rewards usually helps smokers really wanting to quit to successfully stop. Some employers reportedly give employees at least 6 months' notice before implementing the policy.

On-site smoking cessation programs exist most commonly in large companies (more than 1,000 employees), but they have better success rates in smaller worksites (fewer than 250 employees). Facilitators are easily identified and social relationships within the worksite tend to be stronger in larger, dispersed worksites. In larger worksites, employees from the same department should be placed in the same smoking cessation groups to maintain interpersonal relationships and group cohesiveness. Starting a support group of ex-smokers is often helpful to encourage recent quitters to keep it up.

To help build the business case for covering smoking cessation, a group of health care economists—from Kaiser Permanente's Center for Health Research and the industry group America's Health Insurance Plans—is making available online a new modeling tool to help health plans determine how quickly they will see a payoff. The model is based on a recent study that showed financial benefits from smoking cessation programs come in as little as 2 years. Researchers examined 6 years of medical data from 200,000 Kaiser Permanente Northwest members to determine the impact of common antismoking interventions—basically having a doctor recommend and advise in quitting either alone or in conjunction with counseling, nicotine replacement therapy, or other medication. The researchers concluded that modest investments of just $.18 to $.79 per plan member each month began to save money after 2 years. After 5 years, a net monthly cost savings between $1.70 and $2.20 per member existed.

This research is likely to better justify making an investment in smoking cessation because most people stay in a health plan for at least 3 years.

By examining the demographics of your organization and reviewing health risk appraisal data, you can compare your workforce's smoking rate and note whether the subgroups mentioned earlier match your experience; consequently, you can then decide whether to apply the percentage rate by the respective subgroups.

*The three general elements of a successful intervention program are*

1. consistent and repeated advice from a team of supporters to quit smoking,
2. setting a specific date, and
3. providing follow-up visits.

*Additional modalities specifically for physicians include the following:*

- Support and mention of current programs offered at the worksite or in conjunction with the health care provider organization
- Referral to community group counseling
- Advice from more than one clinician (if available)
- Using chart reminders to identify those who smoke

Interventions provided at the worksite or by the health care organization should contain the option of three core elements. A combination of these three elements may not be the best for all smokers; however, to increase the probability of gaining a higher success and reduced relapse rate, the combination of these three strategies should be considered.

The first strategy centers on education and counseling. The education component should focus on the health effects of smoking, the importance of gaining support at work and at home, and moving the individual to the action phase (e.g., setting a quit date). Once an individual is in the action phase, the counselor should work through the following priorities:

- Build readiness to quit.
- Build support needed to quit.
- Build skills needed to quit.
- Identify a quit date.
- Assess success at various time intervals (depending on the client) after quit date.
- Prevent relapse.

The second strategy centers on nicotine replacement therapy (NRT). Once the quit date arrives, the participant should use an NRT such as nicotine gum or a nicotine patch in combination with counseling. When used correctly and in combination with education and counseling, nicotine replacement products increase long-term smoking cessation rates by about one third. Consequently, NRT quit rates around 30% are commonly reported, especially with combined interventions. Overall, a 4-milligram (mg) dose of the nicotine replacement product seems to be more effective than the 2-mg dose in highly nicotine-dependent persons. The evidence suggests that nicotine replacement products are most effective in combination with continuous counseling (Fichtenburg & Glantz, 2002). Users should receive proper instruction on how to use these products as part of the ongoing counseling.

At this time, limited evidence exists that a third type of intervention strategy (non-nicotine prescription drugs) should be used in combination with the education, counseling, and nicotine replacement strategies. The third strategy centers on a brand of sustained-release tablets (Zyban), a non-nicotine aid for smoking cessation. Initially developed and marketed as an antidepressant (Wellbutrin), this drug affects the part of the brain that inhibits addictive behavior. Its effectiveness as an aid for smoking cessation was demonstrated in two placebo-controlled, double-blind trials in nondepressed cigarette smokers. In these studies, Zyban was used in conjunction with individual smoking cessation counseling.

Overall results indicate that Zyban is a successful smoking cessation intervention in approximately 40% of all users.

Self-help programs delivered through the mail and the Internet offer the potential to reach greater numbers of employees and their spouses or partners with cessation treatment. Although the overall effectiveness may be lower than individual- or group-based programs, the overall impact is higher given the greater reach (reach × efficacy = impact). Self-help interventions (written materials in particular) generally produce low initial quit rates, but they are effective in helping quitters sustain their efforts and assisting nonquitters to make additional attempts. For example, the American Lung Association's self-help guide, Freedom From Smoking, and the follow-up version, A Lifetime of Freedom From Smoking, are designed for employees wanting to quit on their own. Self-help kits (e.g., Smoke Stoppers) have produced 1-year quit rates as high as 32%. It is ironic that 81% of current quitters and over 90% of former successful quitters reportedly quit on their own without quitting aids.

Internet smoking cessation programs are growing and have reported varying quit rates. Preliminary research from specific smoking cessation Web sites shows that the quit rate achieved through Internet-based programs may be just as high as traditional, face-to-face programs, but they have not been evaluated rigorously enough to render reliable quit-rate estimates. However, some preliminary, uncontrolled studies of a highly used site (QuitNet.com) show a 3-month quit rate of approximately 7%.

Group cessation methods (multicomponent, behavior-based programs) may produce 1-year quit rates of 30% to 40% but often attract a small percentage of employees. In contrast, incentive- and competition-based programs may attract good participation and produce more favorable quit rates; however, these programs are typically based on self-reported behavior that should be verified with biochemical measures such as thiocyanate or carbon monoxide testing. In a survey of over 200 adult smokers, respondents preferred smoking cessation programs that included

- ways to remain free of smoking for life,
- an endorsement by doctors,
- ways to deal with potential weight gain,
- a list of relaxation techniques to use while quitting, and
- a list of healthy substitutes for smoking.

When evaluating the impact of worksite smoking cessation programs, it is important to define *quit rate, long-term abstinence,* and any other key terms or concepts that can be subjectively quantified. Quit rate is commonly defined as a percentage or ratio of the number of successful employees quitting to the number of employees who started the intervention. A minimum period of 1 year is generally accepted for judging long-term abstinence. Also, be wary of vendors and proposals promising quit rates of more than 40%. Ask vendors for the names and phone numbers of past and current clients who can verify claims.

## Sample Schedule for Implementing a Smoke-Free Policy

Following is an overview of a step-by-step plan for organizations wanting to expand a partial restriction policy into a total smoke-free environmental policy.

• *Months 1 through 3.* In the first month, form a smoking issues committee consisting of managers and labor representatives who are nonsmokers, smokers, and ex-smokers. Consider hiring an outside consultant to facilitate committee meetings and various phases of the project. In months 2 and 3, study the smoking issue by reviewing the company's current policies; other companies' policies; local, state, and provincial ordinances; federal laws (e.g., EPA and OSHA); and legal liability implications with a corporate attorney.

• *Months 4 through 5.* In the fourth month, assess employee attitudes and behaviors relevant to smoking. Develop a simple questionnaire to assess employees' smoking status, attitudes toward the current policy, and recommendations to expand the policy. An easy six-point number scale could be used:

1. Smoking permitted in all areas
2. Designate several smoking areas
3. Designate one smoking area
4. Ban smoking indoors
5. Completely smoke-free workplace
6. No smokers hired (a policy prohibited in some states)

During the fifth month, develop a draft of the proposed policy. Review employee responses, and construct a policy for a preliminary review by senior management. If the policy is not accepted, revise it accordingly, then resubmit it.

• *Months 6 through 9.* Use the sixth month to obtain mainstream support. Meet with key supervisors and middle managers to inform them of the policy and to encourage their support. Announce the new policy in the seventh month by sending a memo from the human resources

### Impact of Worksite Programs—Smoking Control

These examples from well-known companies illustrate potential benefits of smoking control programs and policies.

• **Speedcall Corporation (Hayward, CA):** After the company's president offered each employee a $7 weekly bonus for not smoking at the worksite, the number of smoking employees dropped from 24 to 5 within a year.

• **Dow Chemical (Texas Division):** Twenty-four percent of the company's smokers competed in a smoking cessation competition. Those quitting for at least 1 year entered a raffle for a fishing boat. At prize time, nearly 80% of the entrants had quit smoking.

• **Japan:** A radiator manufacturing company used a multifaceted approach consisting of individualized physician counseling, periodic motivational visits by the occupational health nurse, leaflet distribution, and group discussion. Overall, smoking rates dropped between 8.4% and 12.9% at two follow-up impact evaluations (Kadowaki and Kanda, 2006).

• **UNUM Life Insurance Company (Portland, ME):** The company reported an estimated health care cost savings of $200,000 in the first year of its worksite smoking ban.

• **Pacific Bell (Seattle, WA):** The percentage of smoking employees dropped from 28% to 20% within 2 years of its worksite smoking ban. Visits to the company's health clinic for respiratory problems dropped 13%, and respiratory absences dropped 20%. Collectively, productivity and medical care cost savings exceeded $500,000.

or personnel department to inform all employees of the purpose of the policy and the dates it will gradually go into effect.

• *Months 8 through 9.* During the eighth month, implement partial restrictions to reflect the locations cited in the survey. For example, restrict smoking to designated break areas only. This is also a good time to remove all cigarette machines from the worksite. Devote the ninth month to educating employees on the hazards and costs of smoking. Use various communication methods (e.g., newsletter, message boards, health fairs) to inform employees of the health risks and financial costs of smoking.

• *Months 10 through 12.* Over the next 3 months, begin to offer smoking cessation programs to interested employees and spouses. Review the section on program and policy planning earlier in the chapter to determine appropriate interventions, participation fee policy, program schedules, and incentives. Now is a time to send a memo to all employees outlining the entire policy and reminding them of the dates the policy will go into effect. The policy can now be implemented with clearly defined protocols on monitoring. Schedule monthly meetings over the next 6 months to solicit committee members' feedback on the new policy.

# AIDS EDUCATION AND HIV DISEASE PREVENTION

Acquired Immunodeficiency Syndrome (AIDS) is a growing problem throughout the world. The World Health Organization (WHO) estimates that several million adults are infected with HIV (Human Immunodeficiency Virus). Although men are stricken in greater numbers, women are contracting HIV at a proportionately higher rate. The Centers for Disease Control and Prevention (CDC) estimates that 1 of every 260 Americans has HIV, so it is likely that many American worksites have at least one employee who is HIV positive. Workers in health care settings dealing with body fluids are particularly at risk. Thus, such facilities have developed regulations in response to Healthy People 2010, which stipulates that regulations to protect workers from exposure to blood-borne infections, including HIV infection, should extend to all facilities where workers are at risk of occupational transmission of HIV.

Until the early 1990s, the average life expectancy of a person with HIV/AIDS was projected to be about 2 years (Stine, 1995). According to the CDC, the estimated cost of "lifetime" hospital care for an infected individual can be more than $60,000, and even more for total health care costs. However, medical treatment for persons with HIV disease is steadily improving, enhancing the quality of life for those diagnosed with the disease. In fact, HIV disease is gradually changing from being considered a terminal illness to being viewed as a chronic, treatable illness, at least in some cases. Thus, the increasing number of people who are currently living with HIV disease will live longer and, in many cases, continue to work. Consequently, employers are paying more HIV/AIDS-related costs for medical care and disability pay.

Some employers are already feeling the crunch of HIV/AIDS through higher insurance costs associated with HIV-related claims. In fact, productivity losses from HIV-related illnesses and premature deaths is more than $125 billion a year in the United States alone. Nonetheless, HIV-related health care costs still contribute far less to the nation's rising health care cost index than other factors such as cost shifting, high technology, medical inflation, higher utilization, and medical malpractice insurance premiums.

Faced with the rising health care costs of HIV/AIDS treatment, more companies and insurers are betting on managed care programs to help slow these cost increases. The key to managed care for HIV disease is to reduce inpatient hospitalization, which is the most expensive component of traditional AIDS care. Case management (individualized care at home or in an outpatient facility) is the most common type of managed care used in treating HIV disease; according to some insurers, it is capable of saving as much as $50,000 per case. Furthermore, home care treatment is less expensive, more psychologically comforting, and less likely to expose the patient to other infectious agents that exist in a hospital setting. This type of managed care approach certainly merits consideration as a cost-control strategy. Yet, to effectively deal with this complex and evolving phenomenon, companies will have to establish employee education and prevention activities that appeal to as many employees as possible, especially to those in greatest need.

To date, numerous companies, including Syntex, Bank of America, AT&T, Eaton, Transamerica, and Pacific Telesis, have developed specific personnel policies to deal with HIV disease in the workplace. Bank of America is one of the most progressive companies in this area; it makes certain accommodations (flexible work hours, for example) for an employee with HIV disease, as long as the person's condition does not impair the department's efficiency. Another progressive step is treating HIV/AIDS as any other serious disease and allowing an infected employee to work as long as health permits.

During the mid- to late 1990s, advances in HIV treatments led to dramatic declines in AIDS-related deaths and slowed the progression from HIV to AIDS. However, in recent years, the rate of decline for both cases and deaths began to slow, and in 1999, the annual number of AIDS cases leveled off, while the decline in AIDS-related deaths has slowed considerably.

Employers should address the issue of HIV infection before the first case is reported at the worksite because the employees' level of objectivity and receptivity is probably the greatest then. Waiting to educate employees on HIV/AIDS issues after a coworker has been infected may only intensify general hysteria throughout a workforce.

Employers who have made a corporate commitment to provide HIV/AIDS education have received favorable response from employees, especially when information and education has been integrated into existing health benefits and internal communications.

The Business Leadership Task Force, composed of 15 major northern California employers, has taken a leadership role in providing HIV/AIDS education at various worksites since 1983. A number of task force members such as AT&T, Bank of America, Chevron, Levi Strauss, Mervyn's Department Stores, Pacific Telesis, and Wells Fargo have developed a videotape, *An Epidemic of Fear,* for use in corporate HIV/AIDS information and education campaigns. In addition, several task force member companies provide the following:

- Lectures for managers by HIV/AIDS experts
- Information classes for employees, workers with HIV, and their relatives

## Responding to AIDS: Ten Principles for the Workplace

The Citizens' Commission on AIDS for New York City and northern New Jersey has drafted guidelines to help employers manage AIDS in the workplace. Responding to AIDS: Ten Principles for the Workplace has been endorsed by more than 370 companies and organizations. The principles are as follows:

1. People with AIDS or HIV infection at any stage are entitled to the same rights and opportunities as people with other serious or life-threatening illnesses.

2. Employment policies must, at a minimum, comply with federal, state, and local laws and regulations.

3. Employment policies should be based on the scientific and epidemiological evidence that people who are HIV positive or who have AIDS cannot transmit the virus to coworkers through ordinary workplace contact.

4. The highest levels of management and union leadership should unequivocally endorse nondiscriminatory employment policies and educational programs about HIV disease.

5. Employers and unions should communicate their support of these policies to workers in simple, clear, and unambiguous terms.

6. Employers should provide employees with sensitive, accurate, and up-to-date information about risk reduction in their personal lives.

7. Employers have a duty to protect the confidentiality of employees' medical information.

8. To prevent work disruption and rejection by coworkers of an employee with AIDS or HIV infection, employers and unions should educate all employees before such an incident occurs and as needed thereafter.

9. Employers should not require HIV screening as part of preemployment or general workplace physical examinations, but they can provide the phone number and location of local health department anonymous test sites.

10. In those special occupational settings where a potential risk of exposure to HIV may exist—for example, health care workers who may be exposed to blood or blood products—employers should provide specific, ongoing education and training in universal blood and body fluid precautions as well as the necessary equipment to reinforce appropriate infection-control procedures.

- HIV/AIDS-related articles in company newsletters
- Video presentations that employees may borrow for home viewing

Although various approaches are being used at worksites, some experts feel that peer-to-peer education among employees is the most effective approach.

# MEDICAL SELF-CARE AND HEALTH CARE CONSUMERISM

Growing concerns over higher health care costs and greater demand for limited health care services in the past decade have prompted thousands of worksites to develop medical self-care and consumerism programs. This emphasis seems well justified. The average person in the United States sees a doctor about five times a year and takes about seven different prescriptions per year; yet, at least 80% of all outpatient doctor visits for new health problems are essentially unnecessary and could have been treated just as effectively through medical self-care. According to the National Center for Health Statistics, as few as 26 different conditions account for as much as 90% of all physician visits (Cherry & Woodall, 2002). These conditions are the following:

| | |
|---|---|
| Asthma | Fever |
| Backache | Hay fever |
| Bronchitis | Headache |
| Chest pain | Heartburn |
| Cold | Ingrown toenail |
| Cough | Laryngitis |
| Cuts/scrapes | Nausea/vomiting |
| Depression | Premenstrual syndrome |
| Influenza (flu) | Sinusitis |
| Diarrhea | Sore throat |
| Earache | Sports injuries |
| Eczema | Sprains and strains |
| Fatigue | Urinary tract infections |

For maximum impact, medical self-care and consumerism efforts should be directed toward both employees and their dependents; dependents' health care utilization is typically 20% or higher than employee utilization. One of the most common strategies used by employers is distributing resources such as self-care books,

newsletters, and videocassettes at the worksite or mailed to employees' homes. These resources are primarily designed to help individuals do the following:

- Identify when a health problem is a minor condition that can be treated through self-care and when it is a true emergency; approximately 55% of all visits to emergency departments are not urgent (see table 4.3).
- Learn how to use self-care measures to treat minor ailments.
- Compare health care providers on important quality and cost criteria.
- Ask the right questions of their health care providers.

**Table 4.3 Most Common Emergency Department Visits**

| Principal reason for visit | Percent distribution |
|---|---|
| Stomach pain, cramps, and spasms | 6.5 |
| Chest pain and related symptoms | 5.1 |
| Fever | 4.8 |
| Cough | 2.7 |
| Shortness of breath | 2.7 |
| Headache | 2.6 |
| Back symptoms | 2.5 |
| Throat symptoms | 2.3 |
| Vomiting | 2.2 |
| Pain, not referred to specific body system | 2.0 |
| Lacerations and cuts – upper extremity | 2.0 |
| Motor vehicle accident | 1.6 |
| Earache or ear infection | 1.6 |
| Accident | 1.6 |
| Vertigo – dizziness | 1.4 |
| Injury to head, neck, or face | 1.3 |
| Low-back symptoms | 1.3 |
| Labored breathing | 1.3 |
| Skin rash | 1.2 |
| Nausea | 1.2 |
| Total | 47.8 |
| All other reasons | 52.2 |

From United States Department of Health and Human Services, CDC, National Center for Health Statistic, Number 340, March 18, 2004. *National Hospital Ambulatory Medical Care Survey: 2002 Emergency Department Summary.*

• Understand cost sharing and key features of health insurance (e.g., who pays for what [premium, deductible, and co-payment], what types of alternative health care providers are in the plan).

Reports at worksites using medical self-care and consumer education interventions indicate they are saving $3 or more for every $1 spent on such efforts. Medical self-care interventions operating at many multisite organizations include core communications, such as self-care books, newsletters (from an employer or health plan), educational seminars, Internet-based resources, subject-specific videotapes, and other promotional materials. One of the fastest-growing resources employers use to target and support high-risk individuals is a telephone-based counseling service. This particular type of service is consumer focused, and the goal is to assist individuals in making better health care decisions at home and with their personal health care provider. The telephone service can be part of the targeted high-risk employee process or set up independently with health plan providers. An additional service that will impact program outcomes is to use this system for chronic disease management and disability management. Essentially, the more preventive care and health services are integrated within the organization, the greater the impact. When developing and implementing such services to one or more dispersed sites, many employers have centered their programs on the following topics:

Allergy education

Asthma management

Back care

Customizing your physical exam and blood profile

Diabetes management

Flu and cold home remedies

High blood pressure management

Women's and men's health issues

For greatest impact, it is important to provide visible support and enroll family members into this activity. Partnering with the local health plans at each of the multisite organizations will provide you with local staff support and reduce funding of the program. Regarding the implementation of their medical self-care and consumer education programs, many worksites introduce and promote them on or around the time of their health plan reenrollment. Finally, when an employer customizes these programs around the needs, interests, and educational backgrounds of their employees, they are likely to build a strong employee–employer partnership in the war against rising health care utilization and costs.

## Quaker Oats Health Management Plan

One of the earliest and most successful worksite-based health management programs that included medical self-care and consumerism was implemented by the Quaker Oats Company in the early 1980s. Its integrated plan, which serves as a model for many worksites, includes the following features:

• A company-produced booklet (*Informed Choices*) that helps employees and dependents decide on when to seek health care, how to compare providers on quality and cost criteria, how to select a health care provider, and what questions to ask a provider.

• Financial incentives within a health expense account in which Quaker Oats allocates a fixed amount of money (approximately $500 per year) that employees can use toward their health insurance premium, deductible, or co-payment. Unused money at the end of the year is applied to the following year's allocation.

• Live Well—Be Well, a health promotion program that offers on-site health screenings, seminars, and personal self-enhancement activities. Participants can earn financial rewards for completing a health risk appraisal and adopting healthy lifestyle practices.

Before adopting its integrated approach, Quaker's health care costs rose about 20% a year; since then, Quaker's health care costs have risen an average of about 7% a year.

# FINANCIAL WELLNESS

One of the newest developments in WHP is personal finance education. Responding to employee requests and growing research linking finance and health, health promotion managers are adding a wide variety of financial education initiatives to their programs, including budgeting, college funding, and retirement planning. Although some of these initiatives appeared in a few EAP-related programs in the 1990s, more worksites have expanded the scope of these programs to include a greater emphasis on financial wellness in the past decade. While the links between financial health and overall health may not be as compelling as other WHP areas, a study of 79,070 employees cited finances as second only to work as the leading source of employee stress (Cash, 1996). Respondents with higher stress levels were 2.6 times more likely to experience 5 or more days of absenteeism than employees with low stress levels. Moreover, studies in 1998 and 2001 involving 46,026 employees in various worksites showed stress as one of the strongest predictors of high health care costs.

Because of increased interest in personal finance issues among many employees, financial wellness education has potential benefits for today's WHP programs. For example, the United States has a 401(k) connection. The 401(k) retirement plan may be a good place for you to initiate financial wellness programs for your employees. Currently, only about 50% of employees fully fund their 401(k) plans and one third don't participate at all. This can become a serious problem for some corporations because 401(k) regulations require minimum participation rates. Also, legal experts warn that employees who retire with inadequate retirement funds might sue their employer because they were not adequately informed of the need to make 401(k) plan contributions. Financial education programs at your worksite may be more easily justified if you can show increased 401(k) participation. A second factor worth consideration is the strong potential for high participant interest. According to a survey, funded by the National Institute of Drug Abuse, of 10,308 employees representing nearly 40 organizations, 60% wanted counseling, workshops, or more information regarding finances. Because such a wide range of personal finance topics exists, it is likely that most, if not all, employees would be interested in at least one financial topic if it were marketed properly.

A third factor that compels numerous organizations to offer financial wellness initiatives is that such programs may attract high-risk populations. For example, various surveys conducted by financial wellness program vendors indicate that over 50% of the participants were classified as high-risk individuals; more than one third of these individuals expressed a strong desire to act on their risk factors within the next 30 days after attending financial wellness workshops. Exit surveys indicate that workshops making the money–health connection are likely to motivate participants to take such actions. A fourth potential benefit from offering financial wellness at the worksite relates to attracting underserved populations. Surveys conducted on financial wellness program participants indicate that as many as 35% of attendees report they seldom or never attended other wellness workshops. This number represents a substantial portion of the traditionally underserved population that typically have lower incomes and are highly interested in personal finances.

Administratively, some companies have chosen to offer financial wellness programs outside the realm of an EAP, either as a stand-alone program to attract employees who are interested only in financial wellness or as a marketing strategy to motivate more financial wellness program participants to participate in other WHP programs.

# PROGRAMMING PHILOSOPHY

Many successful WHP programs exist throughout the world. Although some industry insiders contend that the United States has had more of a culture for research and documentation, WHP programs in other countries are equally, if not more, successful because of their supportive worksite cultures. Yet, the means to achieve such outcomes can vary from continent to continent. For example, WHP programs in the United States tend to focus on behavior change, risk-factor identification, and then trying to change the individual. Critics of this approach contend that building a supportive organizational culture and environment are often sacrificed for short-term results. In contrast, European and Japanese companies are more notorious for building supportive environments—at the worksite and community level—that provide ongoing incentives and opportunities for personal health enhancement. Consider, for example, the famed

North Karelia (Finland) case study in which a communitywide initiative involving schools, worksites, and community groups resulted in a significant decrease of heart disease throughout the Finnish population.

Traditionally, WHP efforts have focused primarily on attempting to control or eliminate risk factors for disease. Health professionals identify unhealthy habits and try to motivate employees to replace unhealthy habits with healthier ones. Employees are encouraged to join behavior- change programs that reward them for changing their behaviors, and subsequently they are told they will decrease their chances of contracting certain diseases and dying prematurely if they do so. The science behind this approach to health promotion is the biomedical model of health and disease that has its roots in the Scientific Revolution of the 17th century. A growing number of health promotion authorities are challenging this traditional approach of health promotion characterized by disease focus, fear, and behavioral control. One of the leading authorities in this movement is Jon Robison, PhD, who has written extensively on the evolving field of holistic health. Dr. Robison contends that in moving from a biomedical model of health promotion to a more holistic model, the focus of health promotion should be on the relationship among the spiritual, biological, psychological, and social dimensions of the human experience that are critical to a true understanding of health and healing. In their book, *The Spirit and Science of Holistic Health,* Dr. Robison and coauthor Karen Carrier provide a definitive and thought-provoking look at holistic health promotion and offer compelling reasons for reinventing health promotion in the modern age (Robison & Carrier, 2004).

Shifting the focus of traditional health promotion to a more holistic approach essentially means more emphasis can be placed on the supportive factors for one's overall health and happiness, not just risk factors for illness and disease. These supportive factors relate to various dimensions that include biological, psychological, emotional, spiritual, financial, intellectual, and environmental attributes.

By recognizing the significant role that spirituality exerts in a person's health, various WHP programs have incorporated the spiritual dimension of wellness into their respective programs. For example, the United States Postal Service was one of the first organizations to do so in the early 1990s by offering a lecture series, "Roadblocks on the Human Path," including Creative Anger Management, Prolonged Grieving, and the Art of Forgiveness. WHP staff members at Mercy Hospital in Mason, Iowa, offer numerous seminars in stress and spirituality, "Spiritual Appetizer" breaks (visualization, meditation, and back-to-nature programs). And Conoco Oil in Houston, Texas, continues to offer a balance of mind–body–spirit programs as well as various theme days, including Random Acts of Kindness Day, Attitude of Gratitude Day, Earth Day, An Ounce of Patience Day, and Serenity Day (based on the Serenity Prayer).

In summary, in order to make sound programming decisions, take time to understand the needs of your population, assess your resources, and determine what types of incentives, activities, and ongoing programs will yield the highest employee and organizational health management dividends. Financial resources are also a major factor to consider in programming decisions. Chapter 5 provides some insights on how to make the most of these resources.

## WHAT WOULD YOU DO?

You have just completed a survey of over 100 corporate clients for your employer, a large managed care company. The survey was designed to assess what types of WHP programs each client would prefer to receive from your staff. Approximately 40% of the clients expressed interest in a traditional offering of health fairs, a walking program, and group lunch-and-learn sessions. The remaining 60% of clients prefer

more individual-based and spirit-enhancement offerings. Despite the contrasting preferences, your WHP colleagues prefer the "one size fits all" philosophy and are leaning toward offering the traditional entrée to all clients. However, you would like to tailor WHP offerings to each client's preference despite knowing that it will cost your organization more up front to do so. Aside from the issue of customer satisfaction,

SELECTING HEALTHY LIFESTYLE PROGRAMS  • • •  **59**

what other factors should the WHP staff consider before opting for their approach or your approach? Does any research suggest that one approach is best in meeting employees' health and organizational health status? Where does your boss stand on this issue? Many questions evolve the more you think about your options. What would you do?

# Undertaking Financial Preparations

---

## LEARNING OBJECTIVES

After reading this chapter you will be able to

→ Identify several ways in which to fund a WHP program.

→ Compare potential advantages and disadvantages of an integrated WHP program.

→ List the major components of a proposal.

→ Describe the major steps used in preparing a break-even analysis.

---

Some of the most important decisions in getting WHP programs under way involve identifying and using appropriate financial resources. This chapter addresses financial and program funding considerations in making wise use of your resource allocations. In most programming settings, these considerations center on selecting appropriate personnel, equipment, outsourcing options, program budgeting, and integrating cost factors into a proposal. In considering each of these issues, it is important to review your program's vision, mission, and goals to ensure that sound and realistic financial decisions are made throughout all phases of program planning and implementation.

## ALLOCATING RESOURCES

Resources are a major factor influencing the scope and specificity of an organization's WHP. On-site facilities, personnel, and communication resources are only a few of the valuable entities needed to plan and operate a successful program.

## Location

In many worksites, health promotion programs and activities do not have to be confined to a single location. However, an organization's primary goals and resources largely influence the types of programs that can be feasibly implemented. Issues such as operational costs and program effectiveness are influenced to some extent by site selection. In general, if an organization is more interested in keeping costs to an absolute minimum than achieving a high level of effectiveness, it should assess the prospect of conducting programs and activities at off-site facilities. However, if effectiveness is most important to the organization, then it will probably benefit most from on-site programs, especially if the company has more than 500 employees. By and large, the location should be conducive to the structure, function, and goals of each program. For example, will any type of health status assessment or fitness screening be conducted? Will any formal instruction occur? Will participants be seated, standing, or active? What amount of time for daily or weekly participation is needed for participants to achieve their goals? Will audiovisual materials be used? How much space is needed? Is privacy an issue?

Seminar-type programs such as stress management, nutrition, weight management, medical self-care, and smoking cessation are best provided in quiet, classroom-type settings with no distractions. Conference rooms, employee lounges, and cafeterias at low-usage times are also popular locations to offer such programs. For example, Sentry Corporation in Stevens Point, Wisconsin converted an unused area into a "quiet room" specially equipped with sofas, soft lights, and soothing music for employees to ease their stress.

Efficient use of space is particularly important for worksites with limited facilities. First, the worksite should be assessed to determine possible areas for better use. A feasibility grid, such as the one shown in table 5.1, can help planners determine the most efficient use of existing resources. The key is not just to use space that is already used more efficiently but also to take advantage of unused space and accommodating times.

Some smaller companies pool their finances to rent or lease a community fitness center, school gymnasium, or other facility for employee health programs. Other off-site options for employers to consider are commercial health clubs and fitness centers in shopping malls.

## Personnel

The essence of every successful worksite health promotion program lies in the quality of its personnel. You will encounter wide variation in how much responsibility and how large a budget you are given, depending on the size of your

**Table 5.1  Sample Feasibility Grid Framework**

| | AREAS | | | | |
| Activity | Conference room | Cafeteria | Warehouse or outside | Fitness center | Medical center |
| --- | --- | --- | --- | --- | --- |
| Health screening | | | | ✓ | ✓ |
| Health Risk Appraisal | | ✓ | | | |
| **PROGRAMS** | | | | | |
| Physical fitness | | ✓ | ✓ | ✓ | |
| • Walking | | | ✓ | ✓ | |
| • Recreation | | | | ✓ | |
| • Physical therapy | | | | ✓ | ✓ |
| Nutrition and weight control | ✓ | ✓ | | | |
| Back health | ✓ | | ✓ | ✓ | |
| Prenatal health | ✓ | ✓ | | ✓ | ✓ |
| Smoking control | ✓ | ✓ | | | |
| AIDS education and HIV disease prevention | ✓ | | | | |
| Medical self-care and health care consumerism | ✓ | ✓ | | | |
| Occupational injury | ✓ | | ✓ | ✓ | |
| Employee assistance program (EAP) and quality of work life (QWL) | | | | | |
| Stress management | ✓ | | | ✓ | |

company and your position within it. Given the programs determined by the task force through the identification and assessment phases, what types of personnel are needed to implement the program? If the company is large, the task force can examine the issue of whether more professional staff is needed or is affordable. For example, depending on the budget, one of your options is to support an existing staff member in obtaining the desirable skills and additional certifications (see chapter 10).

Because smaller companies must do with little or no professional staff and rely on volunteers or outsourced personnel, can existing personnel be identified to fill some of this gap? Does anyone in the company have health-related expertise? For example, some small companies establish reciprocal relationships with local colleges or universities (e.g., a selected employee can obtain a tuition waiver for specific courses in exchange for the business sponsoring a part-time or full-time internship for college students).

Whether an organization chooses to use professional staff, rely on in-house volunteers, or use a combination approach, it is important for staff members to work together as a team to reach as many employees as possible.

## Consultants and Independent Contractors

As many worksites continue to experience downsizing, aging workers, and greater efficiency demands, many employers call upon local vendors or health promotion consultants to assist them in one or more of the capacities shown on page 64.

Because few organizations really know about a provider's capabilities until a project is actually under way, selecting a vendor or consultant should be approached with a great deal of consideration to ensure a proper fit between all parties. For example, in selecting a consultant, organizations should do the following:

- Identify why a consultant may be needed.
- Check to see whether all internal resources have been fully tapped and whether an

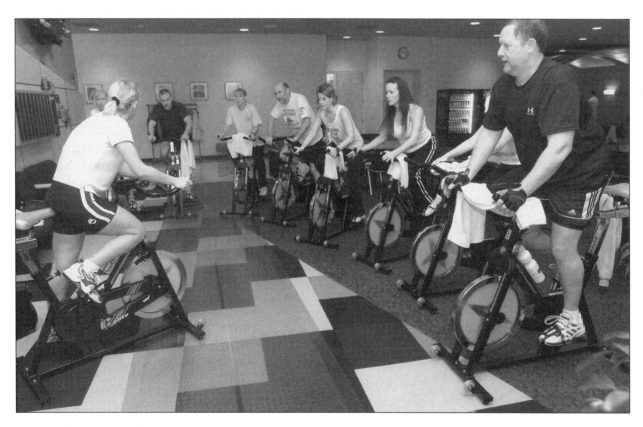

A certified spinning instructor in the workforce or someone who has a strong interest in a particular area that could be tapped for additional training. Would the company pay to get someone certified? Or are there other ways of certification that do not require a substantial investment but that would be just as useful?

## Worksite Health Promotion Consultant Assignments

| Preprogram | Programming | Valuation |
|---|---|---|
| Feasibility studies | Database development | Benefit-cost analysis |
| Risk management | Program planning | Cost-effectiveness analysis |
| Staff development | Incentives design | Break-even analysis |
| Facility design | Marketing | Forecasting |
| Equipment purchase | Integrative operations | Publishing options |
| Health claims | Data analysis | Reengineering |

employee or someone on your staff may be able to solve the problem.

- Solicit bids (detailed proposals) from several consultants.
- Develop a list of criteria to use in judging all candidates. Common criteria include fees, availability, experience, type of clientele served, specialties, opinions of references, and the ability to customize services.
- Thoroughly interview the top candidate(s), and solicit feedback from all staff members.
- Consider the pros and cons of paying a flat fee rather than an hourly fee. Avoid consultants who ask to be paid up front or do not agree to negotiate a specific number of hours.

When an organization uses a consultant or any other resource on a part-time basis, it is important for all parties to clearly understand each entity's role and legal relationship. It is important to avoid any misunderstanding as to what is an employee and what is an independent contractor. The Internal Revenue Service (IRS) applies a standard known as the 20 Factor Test to determine whether workers are employees or independent contractors. The 20 questions are as follows:

1. Do you provide the worker with instructions as to when, where, and how work is performed?
2. Did you train the worker to have the job performed correctly?
3. Are the worker's services a vital part of your company's operations?
4. Is the person prevented from delegating work to others?
5. Is the worker prohibited from hiring, supervising, or paying assistants?
6. Does the worker perform services for you on a regular and continuous basis?
7. Do you set the hours of service for the worker?
8. Does the person work full-time for your company?
9. Does the worker perform duties on your company's premises?
10. Do you control the order and sequence of the work performed?
11. Do you require workers to submit oral or written reports?
12. Do you pay the worker by the hour, week, or month?
13. Do you pay the worker's business and travel expenses?
14. Do you furnish tools or equipment for the worker?
15. Does the worker lack a "significant investment" in tools, equipment, and facilities?
16. Is the worker insulated from suffering a loss as a result of the activities performed for your company?
17. Does the worker perform services solely for your firm?
18. Does the worker not make services available to the general public?
19. Do you have the right to discharge the worker at will?
20. Can the worker end the relationship without incurring any liability?

The IRS considers any "yes" answer to be evidence of an employer–employee relationship that would essentially negate classifying the worker as an independent contractor.

Since the early 1980s, many independent contractors have been hired to work in worksite health and fitness settings because, in large part, such relationships create immediate cost savings to an employer's bottom line. For example, by using an independent contractor, an organization is not required to pay FICA (Federal Insurance Contributions Act, for Social Security), FUTA (federal unemployment), or state unemployment taxes on the worker. In addition, the independent contractor is not eligible to receive company-paid benefits such as health insurance, paid personal leave, disability, vacation, and so on. Typically, independent contractors are not covered by an organization's general liability insurance policy. Thus, the organization should require all independent contractors to carry appropriate liability insurance, show evidence of such current coverage, and make sure the organization is listed as an additional insured on the policy when appropriate.

## Outsourcing

One of the fastest-growing movements influencing today's WHP landscape is outsourcing. Outsourcing is typically referred to as a contract service or "vendor contract." A survey of 927 companies conducted by The Wyatt Company indicates that nearly one third of employers outsource some or all of their human resources and benefits programs. Moreover, many employers continue to outsource their health promotion operations in order to efficiently downsize, focus on their core businesses, and improve their profit margins. Here is a sampling of health promotion and facility management services provided by outside vendors.

Since there are no nationally recognized guidelines to use in selecting community resources, it is important to screen providers, especially those who sell products or services in the following areas: body fat testing, employee assistance program (EAP), preexercise stress testing, nutritional analysis, weight management, smoking cessation, and stress management. Here are some suggested questions to ask and qualifications to check:

1. What types of resources (personnel, money, equipment, and facilities) does the provider have to serve the company's needs?

2. Is the provider certified by a reputable association?

3. Does the provider have a program or service that appears to be philosophically sound and easily understood? Are written goals, objectives, and policies clearly presented?

4. Does the provider have a reasonable fee schedule? Is it willing to offer discounts to firms with small budgets?

5. Does the provider demonstrate substantial expertise in the area? Can it provide a listing of past and current clients?

6. Is the provider willing to provide a complimentary demonstration of the product or service?

7. Can products and services be customized to meet specific needs?

## Commonly Outsourced Health Promotion and Facility Management Services

### Health Promotion Services

Employee health screening
Health promotion seminars
Health fairs
Toll-free self-care services
Health promotion/benefits integration
Health awareness programs
Health information classes
Newsletter publishing
Health risk appraisals

### Facility Management

Preopening promotions and publicity
Conducting a grand opening special event
Hiring, training, and placing fitness staff members
Establishing computerized entry and exit systems
Conduct comprehensive preparticipation fitness evaluations
Supervising all exercise activities
Conducting recreational programs and leagues
Conducting on-site health fairs
Implementing customized incentive programs
Web page design and management

8. Does the provider maintain records in compliance with ADA, HIPAA, OSHA, CDC, etc.?

9. Does the provider have a formal process to evaluate their performance?

## Commercial Health Promotion Materials

In the past decade, many employers have cut their workforces and, thereby, created greater workloads for fewer people. Naturally, this downsizing has created greater pressure on many organizations to stay competitive while using fewer human resources. In response, more organizations are providing their health promotion staff members with health promotion kits, guides, and newsletters to better meet employees' needs. You need to examine both the situations in which you might use such materials and the materials themselves.

Some of the more common arrangements in which these resources are used include the following:

• Large organizations can purchase multiple copies of specific resources to use in hard-to-reach locations or as stand-alone programs where no full-time health promotion staff exists. Multisite operations may have a designated employee at each site acting as a health promotion facilitator to distribute health promotion resources and motivate coworkers to promote their personal health.

• Small businesses can subscribe to multimedia program kits that a designated employee (or outside vendor) can implement on a part-time basis (e.g., take-home videos supplemented with on-the-job stretch breaks)

• Health care provider organizations (e.g., managed care organizations, hospitals, clinics, and public health departments) can conduct actual or adapted versions of these programs at client worksites.

Many employers negotiate arrangements with their health plans to provide health promotion and preventive care services to employees and dependents at designated intervals (e.g., quarterly health fairs). In one nationwide survey conducted by the Center for Corporate Health, nearly all (93%) of the health plans offered members a health newsletter or provided telephone-based advice services. Other activities offered by the health plans include patient counseling and education programs (58%), special prenatal or maternity education programs or materials (81%), and self-care books dealing with prevention or advice on common conditions and complaints for individuals to decide whether to seek medical treatment from a professional or to use self-care (43%). One of the newest examples of how worksites are using their technology networks is the growth of Internet- and intranet-based WHP programs, which employees can access online, 24 hours a day from work or home.

Whether an organization is starting a new WHP or looking for ways to enhance an existing one, it is important to shop around to ensure that the resources selected can be tailored to a particular worksite. For example, assess your target population's needs and interests before purchasing a particular kit or program that may or may not meet your goals and objectives. While some programs are limited to a single topic such as exercise or back health, other programs may provide several topic-specific kits including an array of complimentary resources listed here:

• Educational videos for employees and dependents to view at work and at home; offered bimonthly

• A program announcement memo template that can be e-mailed or otherwise distributed to employees

• A suggested time line for conducting specific phases for implementing certain activities

• A ready-to-use article on a specific topic to reprint in the company newsletter

• Reproducible table tents (folded index cards containing brief health messages placed on cafeteria tables)

• Large two-color program announcement posters

• Small program announcement display posters

• Reproducible handouts and quizzes to motivate employees

• Facilitator guide explaining how to incorporate each kit within a suggested time frame

• Bimonthly facilitator newsletters (tips on implementing certain activities)

• Participant and program evaluation forms

In today's fast-paced, multimedia-oriented world, a wide variety of communication resources are available to WHP personnel. Table 5.2 lists various health education resources to inform,

## Table 5.2  Examples of Health Promotion Communication Tools

| Products and services | COMMUNICATION GOALS | | | | | | |
| --- | --- | --- | --- | --- | --- | --- | --- |
| | Generate awareness | Increase knowledge | Teach skills | Motivate change | Reinforce behavior | Support behavior | Cost per employee |
| Articles | 3 | 3 | 1 | 2 | 2 | 1 | Copy costs |
| Audiotapes | 1 | 3 | 3 | 3 | 3 | 2 | $3-$12 |
| Books and workbooks | 2 | 3 | 3 | 2 | 2 | 1 | $4.25-$12 |
| Booklets | 2 | 3 | 3 | 2 | 2 | 1 | $1.50-$3.75 |
| Brochures | 3 | 3 | 2 | 2 | 3 | 1 | $0.65-$2 |
| Calendars | 3 | 1 | 1 | 2 | 2 | 1 | $3-$9 |
| CD-ROM | 1 | 3 | 3 | 3 | 3 | 1 | $10-$50 |
| Computer programs | 1 | 3 | 3 | 2 | 2 | 1 | $20-$200 |
| Group education programs | 1 | 3 | 3 | 3 | 3 | 3 | $0-$140 |
| Health risk appraisal | 3 | 2 | 2 | 3 | 2 | 2 | $2-$30 |
| Incentives | 1 | 2 | 3 | 3 | 3 | 2 | Varies |
| Interactive video-discs | 1 | 3 | 2 | 3 | 3 | 1 | $50-$100 |
| Internet and intranet | 2 | 3 | 2 | 2 | 2 | 3 | Time to generate or productivity costs |
| Magazines and journals | 3 | 3 | 3 | 3 | 3 | 1 | $1-$2/issue |
| Memos | 2 | 3 | 1 | 3 | 2 | 1 | Copy costs or time to generate |
| Newsletters | 3 | 2 | 2 | 2 | 3 | 2 | $0.20-$0.30/issue |
| One-on-one coaching and counseling | 1 | 3 | 3 | 3 | 3 | 3 | $50 to $125/hr. |
| Paycheck stuffers | 3 | 1 | 1 | 2 | 3 | 1 | $0.15-$0.50 |
| Postcards | 3 | 1 | 1 | 2 | 3 | 1 | $0.15-$0.50 |
| Posters | 3 | 1 | 1 | 2 | 3 | 1 | $1.50-$6.00 |
| Self-help and support groups | 1 | 3 | 3 | 3 | 3 | 3 | Lost production time if done on company time |
| Tabletop displays | 3 | 2 | 1 | 2 | 3 | 1 | $0.50-$1.50 |
| Telephone-based services | 1 | 3 | 3 | 3 | 3 | 3 | $0 to $25 |
| Videotapes | 2 | 3 | 3 | 3 | 3 | 1 | $5-$150 |

Rating: 1 = low impact on communication goals; 2 = moderate impact on communication goals; 3 = high impact on communication goals.

Elin Silveous and George Pfeiffer, printed with permission *Worksite Health,* Winter 1995, pp. 26-27.

educate, motivate, and support employees in their quest for good health. Your choice of tools from this chart depends on a number of variables, including the target group's needs and interests, access to services, and learning style as well as your program goals and objectives, resources, budget, and an analysis of which tools are likely to achieve the greatest return on your investment. Learning style is particularly important to consider in selecting communication resources because people learn in different ways. Thus, you should use various communication tools to reach as many people as possible.

When reviewing the table, avoid the temptation to select only one or two tools that the table indicates will achieve a certain goal. Remember, the most successful WHP programs combine tools to achieve definable results that, when implemented, result in a cohesive intervention strategy, designed to support individual health decisions.

## FUNDING PROGRAMS

For most companies, the decision whether to try a WHP program comes down to funding. Because one of the biggest challenges for a pro-

gram director is to position WHP as an effective strategy to control costs while improving health and well-being among the work staff, the issue of how much it will cost to initiate (or sustain) a WHP program can be a delicate one. Unfortunately, in many work settings WHP programs are viewed as the "new kid on the block" and thus must operate with limited or conditional funding from management. Sometimes program planners can dodge this situation by positioning their programs in places where they will receive more visibility and management support. For instance, in many companies WHP programs are housed in human resources, benefits, personnel, medical, or safety departments. Thus they operate within a single departmental budget rather than on a separate budget. A program may or may not do well under such an arrangement. If, for example, the department within which the WHP program is located experiences an unexpected expense, crucial dollars for funding health promotion may be cut or completely eliminated. This risk is worth taking in the view of many program directors, especially if one can request a separate budget within the department to ensure adequate resources. In any case, the strategy of

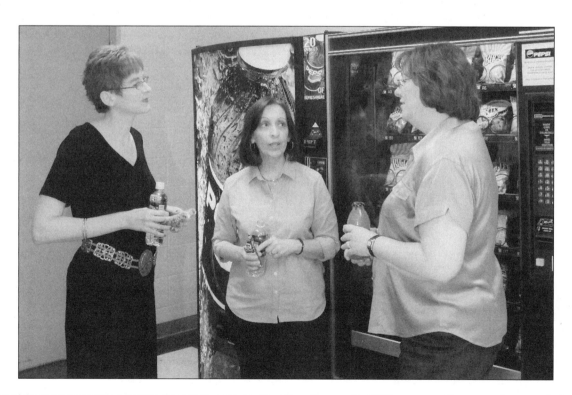

In one of the most innovative schemes, General Dynamics in San Diego finances its WHP program with revenue from on-site food and beverage vending sales. In 1949, the company subcontracted the machines through a nationwide food service company and, in return for reporting repair and servicing needs, receives 18% of the gross vending sales.

receiving greater funding for health programs by integrating them with another department is worth considering.

Some employers try to offset part of the WHP expense by charging employees modest fees for participating in specific programs and activities. For instance, we surveyed several companies with on-site fitness centers and found that annual fees for using the center ranged from $80 to over $500 (most charged between $100 and $200 per year). While some worksites contend that fees are financially necessary and actually boost participation rates, other companies choose not to charge employees fees for programs and activities, hoping that free participation and access will be an incentive.

Several alternative funding strategies that may exist for organizations who wish to look beyond conventional funding arrangements are as follows:

• *Grants.* Numerous organizations offer short-term grants for employers starting new WHP initiatives. You may obtain grant information by contacting your local health department, state health department, regional health associations (such as American Heart Association, American Lung Association, American Diabetes Association, and so on), and federal agencies (such as the Centers for Disease Control and Prevention, National Institutes of Health, National Institute of Environmental Health Sciences, Occupational Safety and Health Administration, and so on).

• *Pooling.* Some worksites, especially smaller employers in a defined geographic area, merge to form a business consortium or pool in which each worksite pays a set fee to a single vendor for selected services (e.g., employee health screening, health fairs, on-site mammography, employee assistance program, and so on).

• *Health plan.* Many worksites, especially mid-size and larger employers, possess the leverage to negotiate discounted WHP programs from their health plan.

These kinds of innovative funding opportunities are available to many companies who have the vision to recognize them.

## PREPARING A BUDGET

Budgeting is one of the most effective ways that WHP decision makers can demonstrate accountability to various stakeholders. In preparing a program budget, WHP directors typically consider key factors such as the following:

• *How others within the organization view WHP.* It is important to gain as much information and insight about how your department, programs, and services fit into the overall mission and goals of the organization. Thus, it pays to regularly review the WHP vision, mission, and goals to see whether they truly reflect the organization's vision, mission, and goals.

• *How recent programs and budgets have performed.* In taking stock of recent activities, it is important to ask key questions. Which programs appear to produce the highest value for the least expense? Could an underachieving program yield greater value with some additional funding or creativity? What piece of the budget should be scrutinized further at regular intervals (e.g., staff, incentives, marketing, evaluation, equipment, and so on)? Either a benefit-cost analysis (BCA) or a cost-effectiveness analysis (CEA)—highlighted in chapter 8—can be a useful tool to help you make these decisions.

• *Using program analysis outcomes.* Head-to-head evaluations of specific programs can be used to create cost projections for each line-item on your budget, such as salaries, equipment purchases, facility operations, marketing, and office supplies.

• *Soliciting input from all staff members.* Expenses for each department should be assessed at regular intervals. Consider using the principles of zero-based budgeting so all department heads are encouraged to think about and justify what they are doing. This type of budgeting requires staff members to build their case for each expense item starting with a zero-based dollar amount.

• *Allowing for flexibility.* It is essential to be flexible when creating a budget to allow for inevitable changes in participation rates, operational cost variations, staff compensation increases, and other fluctuations that distinguish expectations from reality. Thus, it is important to keep notes though out the year to monitor any changes that will help decision makers identify possible reasons for any aberration and make appropriate adjustments in next year's budget.

• *Keeping everything in perspective.* Budgetary control is time consuming. Budget goals are important, but not at the expense of programming goals. For example, is it really worth spending several days to research, analyze, and justify a new $200 program when your total budget exceeds $100,000? A spirit of common sense and practicality will help budget makers maintain a level of objectivity that is crucial for effective budget preparation.

WHP budget makers need to develop a sound proposal for decision makers. A proposal is more likely to be accepted if it includes itemized costs and shows how proposed programs and resources can meet company needs. For example, research conducted by staff members at one worksite showed probable costs for conducting a low-back stretching and flexibility program, as reflected in table 5.3. Based on the comparison shown in the table, the projected benefit ($164,098) exceeds the

### Table 5.3   Direct Cost Items and Projected Benefits of a Prework Stretch Program

| DIRECT COSTS | | | | |
|---|---|---|---|---|
| | Daily | Weekly | Monthly | Yearly |
| *Personnel (program leader)* | | | | |
| Time required (hrs)* | .166 | .666 | 2.66 | 32 |
| Hourly wage ($) | × 15.00 | × 15.00 | × 15.00 | × 15.00 |
| Total personnel cost ($) = | 2.49 | 9.99 | 39.90 | 480 |
| *Productivity (employees)* | | | | |
| Work time for program (hr)* | .166 | .666 | 2.66 | 32 |
| Employees' hourly wage ($) | × 13.50 | × 13.50 | × 13.50 | × 13.50 |
| Number of employees | × 300 | × 300 | × 300 | × 300 |
| Total productivity cost ($) = | 672 | 2,697 | 10,973 | 129,600 |
| *Total personnel and productivity costs* | | | | **$130,080** |
| PROJECTED BENEFITS (1-YEAR IMPACT) | | | | |
| *Health care spending* | | | | |
| Number of employees | 300 | | | |
| Company's back-injury rate last year (15%) | × .15 | | | |
| Number of employees reporting back injury | 45 | | | |
| Average cost per back-injury claim ($) | × 3.015 | | | |
| Total low-back injury claim costs ($) = | 135,675 | | | |
| *Productivity loss* | | | | |
| Number of disability days per back injury | 7.5 | | | |
| Number of back injuries | × 45 | | | |
| Number of back-injury disability days | 337.5 | | | |
| Average productivity loss cost per day** ($) | × 138.24 | | | |
| Total productivity loss cost per year ($) = | 46,656 | | | |
| *Total health care and productivity loss costs* | | | | *$182,331* |
| *Estimated impact of program (90%)**** | | | | *× .90* |
| *Estimated cost-avoidance (benefit)* | | | | *$164,098* |
| *Total personnel and productivity costs* | | | | *-$130,080* |
| *Net savings* | | | | *$34,018* |

*Time required reflects an average of 15 minutes per day for the program facilitator to prepare the worksite and perform the stretching and flexibility routine.

**Based on average hourly compensation (wage of $13.50 per hour and company-paid benefits of $3.78 per hour) multiplied by 8 hours (average workday).

***Based on selected findings reported in the professional literature.

projected program costs ($130,080), suggesting a low-back health program on company time would be a worthy investment.

WHP program developers should determine budgetary needs based on the types of resources required for a new or existing program. In setting up a budget, program planners need to distinguish between variable and fixed expenses so as to forecast appropriately. For example, variable expenses are costs that vary from month to month (e.g., utilities, advertising, certification renewals, and equipment purchases). In contrast, fixed expenses are costs that are consistent throughout the year (e.g., personnel salaries, facility and equipment leasing, and maintenance). Because new programs may require greater start-up expenses for new personnel, staff training, facilities, equipment, and materials, you can use an expense management grid to evaluate budgeting options (see below). In developing a customized grid for a particular worksite, first list the major expense categories for a specific program or activity across the top of the grid. Second, list specific options on the left side of the grid. Third, review the available literature, conduct a survey of the local market, or talk with other worksite health professionals to help you identify major issues. Finally, use all this information to identify possible relationships on the grid. For example, results from a market survey may indicate that it is more time- and cost-effective to hire a local physical therapist to conduct low-back health seminars at a worksite rather than paying to train and certify a staff member for this task.

Because the direct worth of expense items varies from site to site, program planners should consider various options to determine the most efficient way to use specific resources. Some typical questions during this phase include the following:

- Is it more economical for in-house personnel to operate on-site facilities and programs compared to an outside (contract) firm? What is the cost difference?

## Expense Management Grid

List the major expense categories for a specific program or activity across the top of the grid. Then list the specific options on the left side of the grid. Third, review available research, conduct a survey of the local market, or talk with other WHP professionals to help you identify major issues. Finally, use all this information to identify possible relationships on the grid.

### MAJOR EXPENSE CATEGORIES

|  | Personnel | Facilities | Utilities | Equipment | Materials | Advertising | Maintenance |
|---|---|---|---|---|---|---|---|
| Services estimated |  |  |  |  |  |  |  |
| Services negotiated |  |  |  |  |  |  |  |
| Services contracted |  |  |  |  |  |  |  |
| Services donated |  |  |  |  |  |  |  |
| On-site |  |  |  |  |  |  |  |
| Off-site |  |  |  |  |  |  |  |
| Purchase new |  |  |  |  |  |  |  |
| Purchase used |  |  |  |  |  |  |  |
| Donated |  |  |  |  |  |  |  |
| Bid |  |  |  |  |  |  |  |
| Other (list) |  |  |  |  |  |  |  |

- Is new equipment needed, or will used equipment do? If used or leased equipment is suitable, what type of warranty can be obtained? How often will the equipment need to be replaced?
- Will in-house staff have the time and skills to analyze health claims data as quickly, cost-effectively, and objectively as an outside firm?
- Will an in-house EAP be as appealing to employees as an external EAP?
- What kinds of resources may exist at the local university to assist with the WHP efforts?

# PREPARING YOUR PROPOSAL

Once program planners have made key decisions about goal setting, funding and budgeting, and how to manage WHP programs, they are ready to prepare a proposal for management. Presenting the program proposal is a crucial stage in the planning phase. Present the proposal poorly, and the plug may be pulled on the program before it ever has a chance to prove its value.

In preparing a health promotion program proposal, it is essential that it address a company's specific health management needs. Although every proposal will vary according to the unique nature of an organization and its employees, each should contain the following sections:

- Problem identification
- Goal
- Environmental assessment
- Worksite strategies
- Resource assessment
- Proposed program
- Expected costs
- Expected benefits
- Overall benefit-cost projection

For example, assume that a company's health care costs are rising faster than anyone's projections and that a health promotion program is being proposed. Upon reviewing the company's health care claims data, program planners discover that (1) the most common type of health care claim filed by employees is musculoskeletal and (2) low-back injuries are involved in most of these claims. Based on this information, program planners prepare a proposal for a back-injury prevention program (see below).

## Sample Program Proposal

### 1. PROBLEM IDENTIFICATION

Program planners reviewed the company's health care claims and cost data, which revealed the most common claims to be musculoskeletal:

**Table 5.A  Average Cost Per Claim**

| Type | # of claims | Total cost | Average cost/claim |
|---|---|---|---|
| Back injuries | 100 | $65,000 | $650 |
| Knee injuries | 33 | 9,174 | 278 |
| Shoulder injuries | 14 | 1,400 | 100 |

### 2. GOAL

Reduce the number and average cost per claim of musculoskeletal injuries, especially low-back injuries.

### 3. ENVIRONMENTAL ASSESSMENT

Further analysis and worksite observations by on-site personnel indicated the following:

- Employees most affected: 25- to 45-year-old men working in the shipping department.
- Most common time of occurrence: 75% of all low-back injuries occurred in the first 2 hours of the work shift.
- Type of injury: 90% of all back injuries were classified as muscle strains in the low back.

- Activity at time of injury: 60% of all low-back muscle strain injuries occurred while the victims were lifting.

## 4. WORKSITE STRATEGIES

In-house staff members called local employers and reviewed several scientific journal articles on low-back injury prevention programs. They found numerous companies with successful programs, such as the following:

**Table 5.B  What Some Organizations Are Doing to Minimize Back Injuries**

| Company | Program features | Impact |
|---|---|---|
| Biltrite Company (Chelsea, MA) | Employee education Prework stretching | 90% drop in workers' comp costs |
| Capital Wire (Plano, TX) | Prework stretching Employee education | Fewer back injuries; $180,000 saved |
| Lockheed Corporation (Sunnyvale, CA) | Prework stretching Employee seminars | 67.5% drop in back injury costs |

## 5. RESOURCE ASSESSMENT

What types of on-site resources can be used to develop an effective low-back injury prevention program? Staff members conducted an on-site inventory that indicated:

- Available resources
    1. Facility: Large warehouse area
    2. Promotional materials: Employee newsletter
    3. Budget: $1,500 is available in the human resources department discretionary fund
- Needed resources
    1. Equipment: Padded floor mats needed for back and abdominal floor exercises
    2. Incentives: A quarterly sweepstakes program with prizes!!!

## 6. PROPOSED PROGRAM

Based on the health problem identified and available resources, program planners recommend the following program:

### Back Basics: A Worksite Back-Injury Prevention Program

Target Area: Shipping department employees

- *Phase 1 (January): Awareness and publicity.* The number of low-back injuries reported at the worksite will appear in this month's issue of the employee newsletter and be repeated on a quarterly basis. The article will explain the primary reasons for the new program with specific responsibilities for shipping department supervisors, employees, and the occupational health nurse. This information will also be shared during the next safety meeting held on the second and fourth Mondays of each month.
- *Phase 2 (February): Training.* The occupational health nurse will conduct training sessions for all shipping department supervisors and employees during bimonthly safety meetings. Topics will include back anatomy; ergonomic factors; and proper lifting, pulling, and pushing techniques.
- *Phase 3 (March): Incentives.* Worksite posters, newsletter articles, and weekly e-mail messages will describe how to enter the Back Basics Sweepstakes program. All shipping department employees reporting no back injuries in the previous quarter can compete for prizes each quarter.

*(continued)*

- *Phase 4 (March): Implementation.* Shipping department supervisors will lead their respective employee teams through a mandatory back stretching and strengthening routine during the first 5 minutes of their work shift. After the first week, individual employees will assume responsibility for leading daily sessions on a rotating basis.
- *Phase 5 (July): Monitoring and evaluation.* The occupational health nurse will review back-injury data every 6 months to determine the impact of the daily prework routine and the need, if any, to revise the protocol for greater impact in the future.

## 7. EXPECTED COSTS

Based on the identification and needs assessment, program planners estimate that annual operating costs for the proposed program will be as follows:

- Personnel: no additional cost
- Facility: no additional cost (will use existing space)
- Equipment: padded floor mats; $400
- Promotions/sweepstakes prizes: $250 per quarter, or $1,000 per year

Total: $1,400

## 8. EXPECTED BENEFITS

Based on a review of other worksite low-back injury prevention programs, the following benefits are expected to occur within 12 months of the program inception:

| | |
|---|---|
| Fewer job-related back injuries | Greater productivity |
| Fewer back-injury absences | Improved musculoskeletal flexibility |
| Reduced low-back claim costs | Less overtime expenses paid to replacement workers |

## 9. OVERALL BENEFIT-COST PROJECTION

The proposed program is modeled after successful worksite back-injury prevention programs and expected to conservatively produce a minimum 10% impact on designated cost outcomes. For example, the proposed program should reduce the number of projected back injuries from 90 to 81. Because the average cost of one low-back strain is about $1,000, a 10% impact would produce cost savings of approximately $9,000. If two or more injuries are averted during the year, anticipated cost savings would exceed programs costs ($1,400), as shown here:

### Table 5.C  Benefit-Cost Ratio

| Injuries avoided | Benefit | Program cost | Benefit-cost ratio |
|---|---|---|---|
| 9 | $9,000 | $1,400 | 6.43:1 |
| 8 | $8,000 | $1,400 | 5.63:1 |
| 7 | $7,000 | $1,400 | 5.00:1 |
| 6 | $6,000 | $1,400 | 4.28:1 |
| 5 | $5,000 | $1,400 | 3.57:1 |
| 4 | $4,000 | $1,400 | 2.85:1 |
| 3 | $3,000 | $1,400 | 2.14:1 |
| 2 | $2,000 | $1,400 | 1.43:1 |
| 1 | $1,000 | $1,400 | [.71:1] |

Management will presumably consider this proposal because it

1. clearly describes the identified problem,
2. suggests a practical strategy to address the problem, and
3. shows that benefits will probably exceed programming costs.

To be effective, every proposal must meet these three criteria.

While reviewing a proposal, management may want to know when a program or strategy will pay off or break even. For example, assume a company is planning to convert an old warehouse into a fitness center with a two-person staff consisting of a program director and a fitness specialist. By determining specific costs and usage patterns of the fitness center, program planners can develop a break-even analysis. A sample break-even analysis follows.

In using any economic analysis technique, be aware that various factors can jeopardize expected outcomes. In our preceding example, the estimated time frame of 52.5 weeks may be extended by unforeseen or uncontrollable events—if the participation level drops below the expected level, unexpected programming costs are incurred, or if employee wages and benefits or the company's cost to replace absent workers increase faster than absenteeism costs. On the other hand, if participation levels

## Break-Even Analysis for an On-Site Fitness Center

1. Determine start-up costs for converting an existing space (year 1 only):

   Fitness center equipment: $50,000

2. Determine annual fixed costs:

   Maintenance of equipment: $1,000

   Depreciation of equipment: $5,000

3. Determine annual variable costs:

   Program director: $45,000*

   Fitness specialist: $30,000*

   Utilities, office materials, etc.: $4,000

   Program incentives: $3,000

4. Calculate total fixed and variable costs:

   $138,000

5. Determine projected usage rate of fitness center:

   Size of workforce: 1,000 employees

   Percentage of workforce expected to participate × 20% (national average)

   Usage rate: 200 employees

   Number of weekly visits per participant × 2

   Total weekly visits: 400

6. Determine financial benefits from the fitness center visits:

   The desired outcomes will vary from program to program. The outcome variables classified as corporate benefits (cost savings) in this example are reduced absenteeism and lower medical care expenses.

   Corporate benefit per participant: $6.57**

   Number of total weekly participant visits × 400

   Total corporate benefit per week: $2,628

7. Determine break-even point by dividing total cost by financial benefit per week:

   Total costs: $138,000

   Corporate benefit per week: $2,628

   Time of participation needed to break even: 52.5 wk

8. Plot costs and benefits on a time frame (see figure 5.1):

Based on the preceding break-even analysis, the company's fitness center investment is projected to pay for itself ("break even") at the beginning of the second year (between 52 and 53 weeks).

*An annual salary and benefits (compensation) inflation rate of 3% is applied; for example, the program director's first-year salary of $45,000 would be $46,350 in year 2 and the fitness specialist's first-year salary would be $30,900 in year 2.

**Based on research studies showing exercisers (1) are absent at least 1.2 days less than nonexercisers; 1.2 days × $320 = $384 per absence; $384 / 52 weeks = $7.38 / 2 (weekly visits) = $3.69, and (2) incur at least $300 less in annual medical care expenses than nonexercisers; $300 / 52 weeks = $5.77 / 2 (weekly visits) = $2.88 per visit. *Note:* The daily compensation value of $320 is based on a U.S. worker's average wage and benefits of $20 per hour: $20 × 8 hours = $160 daily compensation paid to an absent worker and a replacement worker.

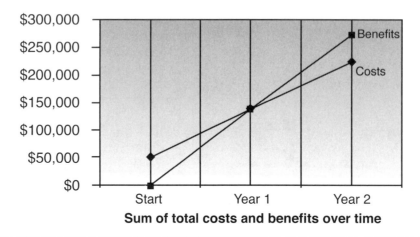

**Figure 5.1**  Sample break-even analysis plot.

exceed the expected level, participant absenteeism drops, or wages and replacement costs increase more slowly than absenteeism costs, then the break-even point would occur before 52.5 weeks.

Once the program has been proposed to and accepted by management, the program planner is nearly ready to implement the program. However, two more steps are necessary before the program can be safely launched: screening employees for health risks and giving the program a trial run. These steps are described in chapter 7.

## POSITIONING WHP IN AN INTEGRATED FRAMEWORK

Since the mid-1990s, a growing number of worksites have developed an integrated health management approach to enhance employee health, safety, productivity, and morale. In fact, various studies on organizational frameworks and cost-control efforts of many companies have shown a direct relationship between integrated health management and cost control. As a group, companies operating an integrated approach showed average health care cost increases approximately one third less than the national average. This decisive cost-control advantage enables these companies to invest more money in research and development, employee training, and employee incentives to enhance their long-term profitability. Strategies to accomplish this goal include partnering with various groups inside and outside of the worksite. In their quest for integration, employers work to progressively

shift their focus from a traditional focus (e.g., fitness center–based) to addressing the impact of health on productivity, safety, and profitability. These shifts encourage WHP staff to seek out and work with other departments that have expertise that could further impact employee health. This often requires a culture change and a commitment to break down organizational silos of individual interest. Consequently, WHP personnel can partner with others in human resources, benefits, risk management, safety, and medical services to make the transition from cost centers to partners in expense management (see figure 5.2). Such relationships foster real worksite cases of opportunity and success. For example, consider the following situation that actually occurred at an insurance company. An employee on disability for a mental health diagnosis requested a leave of absence as an accommodation. The return-to-work professional identified potential alternatives and requested input from the employee assistance program (EAP). Through that relationship, the employee received counseling and coaching that supported an early return to work and provided improved life skills that the employee continues to use to successfully manage the mental health issues. In another instance, an occupational health nurse conducted a basic health screening on a new employee and detected poor low-back flexibility. Because the nurse was working in an integrated program, she worked with

- human resources to discuss appropriate job tasks within the employee's physical capabilities,

- WHP staff members to develop a personalized back health program to improve the individual's flexibility, and
- safety personnel to educate the new employee on company policies for proper lifting.

Even small employers have shown benefits from an integrated health management framework. The overall success of an integrated health management framework depends largely on an organization's ability to

- develop health management goals that are realistic,
- employ health management personnel with the skills to achieve each goal,

- delegate appropriate personnel to specific goals, and
- establish an operational framework that enhances interpersonal and interdepartmental communication and teamwork.

An integrated approach, though increasing in popularity nationwide, has potential disadvantages as well, the main one involving autonomy. By its nature, an integrated approach depends on teamwork and decision by committee. This can work well, but the decision-making process will likely break down if departmental representatives push their personal agendas. When this occurs, department leaders might become frustrated over the inability to arrive at decisions in a timely manner. In some cases, WHP

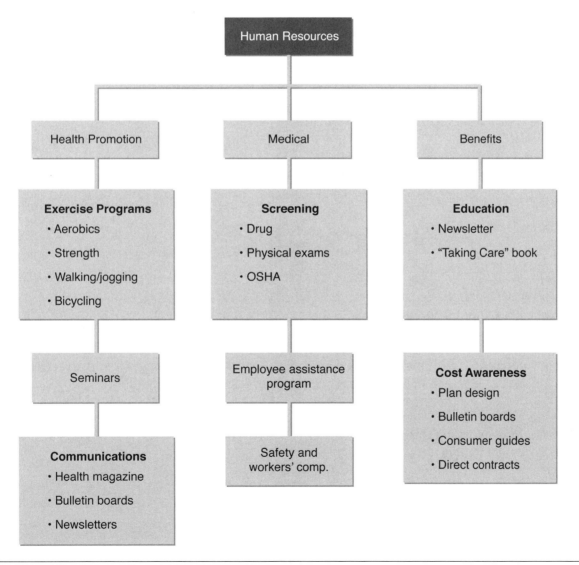

**Figure 5.2** The integrated health management framework used at Lord Corporation.

personnel are discouraged to find out how little clout they have in an integrated approach. In order to minimize these reactions that can lead to wide-scale alienation and personnel fallout, it is important to develop an integrated framework and decision-making protocol that fosters input from all stakeholders. Such efforts obviously require constant monitoring and revisions to factor in personnel, budget, political, and cultural changes that will occur in time.

## Assessing Your Planning Efforts

As you proceed from the program planning phase to creating a healthy worksite culture (discussed in chapter 6), check to see whether your planning efforts have created specific standards for success. For example, check to see whether your planning efforts have generated the following:

- Commitment from senior management to dedicate sufficient resources—funding, personnel time, equipment, and facilities. Ideally, management also shows support by participating in the program.

- A clear statement of philosophy, purpose, and goals that declares the organization's commitment to motivate and assist a significant portion of employees to practice healthier lifestyles.

- A process for assessing organizational and individual needs, interests, risks, and costs.

- Leadership from well-qualified, health promotion professionals in the program's design, implementation, and ongoing operations.

- A program design that addresses the most significant health risks, specific risks within the employee population, and needs of the organization.

- High-quality programs that motivate participants to achieve lasting behavior changes and higher quality of life.

- Effective marketing to achieve and maintain high participation rates.

- Efficient systems for program operation and administration.

- Evaluation procedures for assessing program quality and outcomes.

- A system of communication for sharing program results with employees, staff, and senior management.

## WHAT WOULD YOU DO?

Suppose you work for a company that has never had WHP. Management has asked you to design and implement a new medical self-care program for employees. Your research efforts show that the most effective intervention is voluntary and consists of self-care books, financial incentives, and quarterly on-site seminars. You learn that this program can yield as much as a $4 benefit for every $1 spent. However, the research suggests that a participation rate of 50% for at least a year is necessary to achieve a positive benefit-cost ratio. Your worksite is currently downsizing, and management expects you to show a positive return within 6 months. In preparing your proposal for the new program, what should you do to achieve management's goal within the shorter time frame? Should you propose a mandatory program to ensure 100% participation? If not, should you recommend higher financial incentives to motivate a high rate of voluntary participation? Should you offer a higher number of on-site seminars? Describe and justify your strategy.

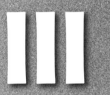

P A R T

III

# Accomplishing and Evaluating Worksite Health Promotion

# Reducing Major Health Risks

After reading this chapter you will be able to

→ Describe several ways that an employer can provide a healthy worksite.

→ Explain why employers should assess the risk of cumulative trauma disorders in the workforce and introduce several prevention strategies.

→ Identify several factors an employer should consider before establishing an Employee Assistance Program (EAP).

→ List several ways an employer can create a less stressful worksite environment.

O ne of the biggest challenges facing employers is reducing major health risks among employees. Much of their success will hinge on the extent to which they can prevent injuries, develop a positive worksite culture in which health is valued, maintain an assistance program for employees to turn to when necessary, and help employees manage the daily stress they encounter at work. In this chapter we discuss various ways of dealing with the work-related issues of creating a healthy worksite.

A question all employers and WHP program directors need to ask is, Does our worksite promote healthy or unhealthy behaviors? For example, take these three worksites: One permits cigarette smoking anywhere in the worksite, the second restricts smoking to certain areas, and the third bans smoking completely. The cultural norm (i.e., expected behavior) in the first company is that smoking is acceptable behavior while the norm in the third company is that smoking is not acceptable, at least not at the worksite. Which of these norms would you want to promote at your worksite?

It should come as no surprise that employees are more motivated to lead healthy lifestyles in a worksite that places a high priority on health. Company policies that do not promote healthy lifestyles should be reconsidered and changed. In most cases, change should be gradually phased in so that employees have time (usually a matter of weeks for a minor change and a matter of months for a major change) to adjust to new policies. For example, Nortel and Pacific Bell phased in a series of worksite smoking restrictions over 2 years before fully implementing their comprehensive clean air (smoke-free) policies. Positive responses far outnumbered the negative at both worksites. Before establishing any major changes in policy, management may take a few months to solicit employees' feedback on the proposed change. Yet, in some instances, management may have decided the change is needed and chooses not to solicit employees' opinions on the proposed change. In both cases, a company will usually spend several months educating employees about the need for the proposed change. Depending on the type of program or policy being proposed, a company may choose to introduce it on a trial basis—say, in certain locations or with a particular group of employees—and then expand it to the remainder of the workforce within a designated time frame. (See chapter 4 for a step-by-step process to phase in a clean air policy.)

# STRATEGIES FOR INSPIRING CHANGE

Depending on an organization's culture and goals, an employer or WHP program director can implement various health promotion strategies to promote and reinforce healthy behaviors. Implementing health promotion activities and incentives that integrate individual, environmental, cultural, and organizational values is far more effective than focusing on any one area alone. These strategies might be general or more specific, such as taking an ergonomic approach or emphasizing exercise or education.

Ergonomics is a science concerned with designing and arranging things so that people and things can interact effectively and safely. In WHP, ergonomic strategies involve designing or placing equipment to be used by employees to make each employee's work tasks more efficient or easy. For example, to minimize musculoskel-etal injuries and boost productivity, a worksite might purchase state-of-the-art office equipment (e.g., custom chairs that adjust to suit each employee's body shape and physical needs) that minimizes risk of overuse injuries.

Some employees appreciate the opportunity to exercise as an end in itself, for the pure enjoyment of it. It so happens that while they are enjoying the physical exertion, they are also becoming more productive and healthy. Here are some ideas for initiating exercise strategies at the worksite:

- Post "point of decision" prompts at key locations to encourage physical activity (e.g., "Take a Few Steps to Better Health" signage in stairwells to encourage stair climbing instead of taking an elevator).

- Set up a free-weights area in the fitness center, a popular feature for bodybuilders and competitive weightlifters.

- Offer gentle fitness classes (combining yoga, low-impact aerobics, and relaxation techniques); intended for all fitness levels, but appeals particularly to employees who are new exercisers or have special physical

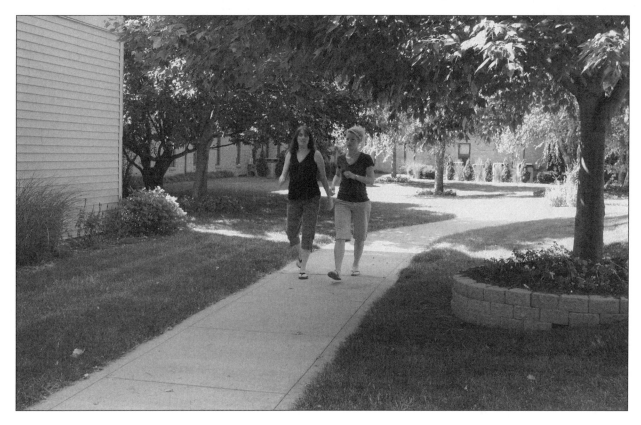

Developing trails near the worksite and encouraging employees to walk or jog during lunch and break times is one type of exercise strategy.

challenges (e.g., back pain, arthritis, muscle stiffness and soreness).

- Provide selected pieces of exercise equipment in suitable locations for employees to use during breaks and lunchtime.
- Encourage employees who sit a lot to take a stretch break for better circulation and work efficiency.
- Equip a designated break area with basketball hoops, table tennis equipment, horseshoe pitching stations, boxing bags, and other recreational equipment.
- Offer discounts or subsidies for fitness club memberships.
- Provide showers and changing facilities for people who exercise at work.
- Create departmental competitions to reward teams with substantial exercise levels each month; if competitions contradict the philosophy of the WHP program, sponsor individual promotions and reward behaviors rather than outcomes.

Nutrition-oriented strategies can be positioned to complement the preceding exercise strategies in helping employees achieve greater health and productivity outcomes. Here are some ways to motivate employees to eat healthier:

- Offer lunch-and-learn sessions in the company's cafeteria on a regular basis. (Explore the prospect of offering these sessions on paid time or extending the designated lunch period for attendees. Consider videotaping these sessions and making them available for checkout.)
- Organize a healthy potluck, including a healthy recipe exchange.
- Gradually change vending machine items to healthy foods and snacks.
- Offer fruit and vegetable snacks instead of junk food at meetings, in common areas, and in break rooms.
- Place table tents with monthly nutrition tips on cafeteria tables.
- Provide employees with coupons, subsidies, or discounts for purchasing healthy meals either at worksite cafeterias or at restaurants and stores that are located close to workplaces.
- Subsidize or discount the cost of heart-healthy entrée offerings in the company cafeteria.

Some employers may choose to offer employees on-the-job opportunities to educate themselves on health issues. Other companies may choose to provide employees with informative materials to take home to read if they choose. While it's more likely that employees may take advantage of on-the-job educational opportunities rather than on their own time, in many worksites it may not be feasible or practical to encourage employees to read on the job (except during lunchtime or on breaks). Here are some educational strategies to make material available to employees; not all of them will be appropriate at every worksite:

- Create and maintain bulletin boards on health information and self-development tips in high-density areas.
- Create a library of books, videos, and audio cassettes for employees to check out or peruse on-site.
- Stock a cart with health magazines, books, and brochures. Periodically move the cart to different locations throughout the worksite.
- Place health magazine racks in bathroom stalls.
- Include a personal health column in the company newsletter.
- Send a daily health message or personal health tip through e-mail to all employees.
- Ask participating employees to write worksite health program testimonial and endorsement letters in the company newsletter.
- Subscribe to a monthly health promotion newsletter for employees to read and share with family members.

Along with the preceding ergonomic, exercise, and educational strategies, here are some more general tactics employers might try to promote healthy practices at the worksite. Some of them are very easy to apply; others will take some time, and you might want to implement them gradually.

- Offer many accessible water fountains or water coolers to encourage employees to drink more water at the worksite. Also, distribute "mail-bites" to inform employees of the benefits of hydration and the fact that most people do not drink enough water each day.
- Convert a 10-by-10-foot area into a "Personal Health Kiosk," a self-contained screening and

## Enhancing the Worksite Environment With a Lactation Program

First National Bank (FNB) in Omaha, Nebraska, is a national leader in providing lactation services to its nursing employees. FNB's worksite includes a lactation suite complete with six private nursing rooms, a refrigerator, a sink, and pumping supplies. Each suite is furnished with a glider rocker, a table, a clock radio, and other amenities designed to make working mothers feel right at home. Security and privacy are highly regarded in the lactation suite. Each nursing mother is issued an access card that allows her to enter the suite, ensuring that only those with current clearance gain entry. Additionally, two outsourced lactation specialists staff the suite, coordinating registration, scheduling, and training. And it's a good thing—the service is becoming more popular with new mothers each year. Best of all, nursing mothers spending time with their babies need not worry about losing work time. Management at FNB decided that time spent in the lactation suite is time well spent, and it does not have to be made up. And working mothers appreciate it.

resource module equipped with an automatic blood pressure cuff, weight scales, health brochures, and other interactive resources.

• Designate a quiet room equipped with comfortable seating and soft music for employees to use in stressful times.

• Designate a period of time for employees to participate in company-sponsored health promotion activities. For example, devote the first 5 minutes of the work shift to stretching exercises, or add 15 minutes to lunch for employees to take a walk.

• Review the company's sick leave policy to determine whether sick days can be renamed to convey a more positive connotation for employees (e.g., personal wellness days).

• Offer employees with excellent attendance a financial bonus or an additional wellness day for each day their absenteeism for a period falls under the company average. (Important note: Work with human resources personnel to ensure that the policy does not discourage employees with real illnesses from seeking necessary health care.)

• Establish smoke-free and safety belt use policies in all company vehicles and facilities.

Building a positive, health-minded culture at the worksite cannot be done in a day—or even in a few days or weeks. The development will take some time and is best done gradually. Programs implemented too quickly often vanish as fast as they appear. Gradual change is much more reliable. A WHP director should never spring large new programs on employees all at once. Small, gradual changes can effectively alter a culture's values whereas big, sweeping changes are usually met with resistance.

Along with developing a work culture that values each person's health and overall well-being, an organization must regularly monitor conditions at the worksite to ensure the facility and equipment are as safe as possible in order to prevent injury. The risk of accidents always exists, but if all stakeholders respond properly to the mishap, the same accident should never occur twice.

## OCCUPATIONAL INJURY

In 1970 the Occupational Safety and Health Act (OSHA) was established to require American employers to provide safe workplaces for their employees. Since then, the incidence of occupational illnesses and injuries as well as the number of lost workdays have decreased substantially (see figure 6.1).

Nearly half of all on-the-job ailments lead to serious work restrictions or lost work time. Moreover, the Social Security Administration predicts that, over the next 10 years, an aging baby-boomer-generation workforce will lead to a 37% increase in the incidence of disability. The most common worksite injuries are cumulative trauma disorders (CTDs), such as low-back strain and carpal tunnel syndrome. These repetitive stress injuries occur over time, usually as a result of performing one or more movements repeatedly day after day.

Cumulative trauma disorders affect approximately 18 million U.S. workers annually. About 2 million of them suffer some degree of carpal tunnel syndrome, 4 million get tendonitis, and about 8.5 million have CTD-related low-back pain. In fact, since 1980, the incidence of CTDs has risen nearly 600%. CTDs now account for

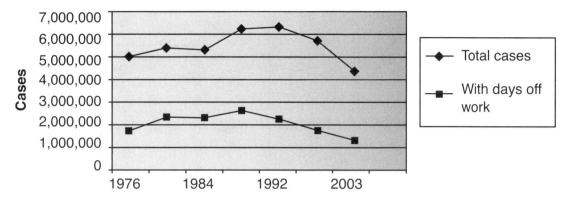

**Figure 6.1** Number of nonfatal occupational injury cases in private industry from 1976 to 2003.

more than half of all workplace injuries (see figure 6.2), and thus no indication exists that this percentage will decrease in the near future. In fact, studies show that about 75% of all American workers will experience a CTD back injury sometime during their working lives.

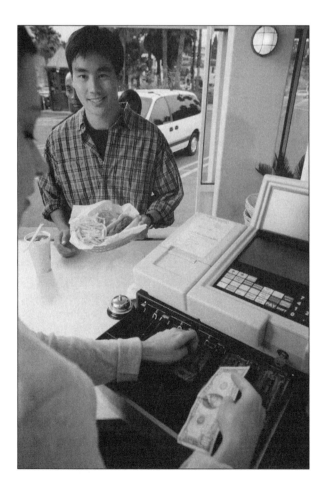

Occupational research indicates that CTDs have affected about 50% of supermarket cashiers, 41% of meatpackers, 40% of newspaper workers, and 22% of telecommunications workers.

What causes CTDs? Various factors may contribute to an employee incurring a CTD, including poorly designed equipment, fast-paced work, few or no rest breaks, stress, poor posture, force and repetition, physical make-up, and poor physical condition. Research suggests that employers are becoming more aware of the costliness of CTDs, which should lead to more care taken in the purchase of supplies. However, the high cost of specially made equipment to reduce CTDs prevents many companies from buying them. According to industry watchers, as more attention is given to the rising costs of CTDs, demand will increase for specialized equipment, resulting in lower prices in the next few years.

## CTD Research

Many studies indicate a positive relationship between reduced injury and specific programs. For example, a study by Canadian researchers investigated the impact of a physical fitness program on job-related injuries and associated costs at a municipal worksite. Each of the 134 participants was tested for back fitness, strength, aerobic power, flexibility, weight, body fat percentage, blood pressure, lifestyle, and productivity. Participants were given an exercise prescription based on their overall fitness level (Sirles, Brown, and Hilyer, 1991). After 6 months of exercising, participants were retested and exhibited a 14.2 % increase in their overall back fitness level. Moreover, injury-related absences dropped one fourth of a day (while nonparticipants' absences increased approximately 3.1 days), producing an estimated cost savings of $62,922. These results resemble those of another study conducted to determine the effect of physical fitness on back injuries in firefighters (Cady, Bischoff, and

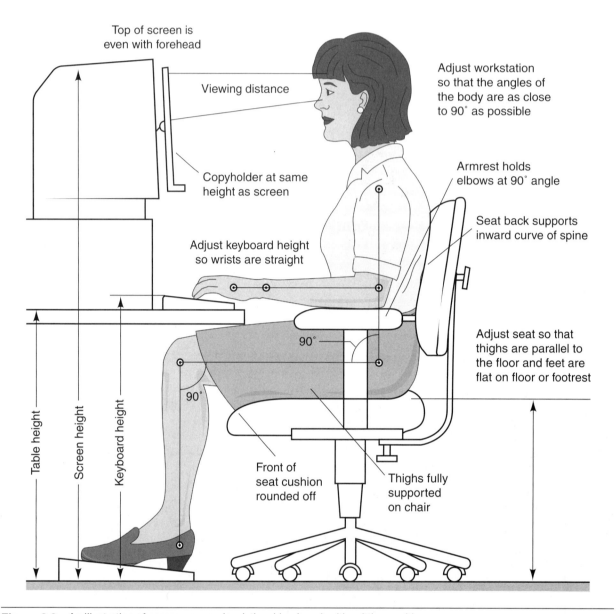

**Figure 6.2** An illustration of proper ergonomic relationships for a healthy sitting position.

O'Connell, 1979). To ensure high fitness levels, the program provided each participant with 3 hours of exercise each week and periodically assessed him or her for the duration of the study. Overall, the study indicated that physical fitness and conditioning prevented back injuries. Moreover, the study showed a statistically significant drop in the number of injuries sustained with a corresponding gain in physical fitness. A follow-up study spanning a period of 14 years showed enhanced fitness levels strongly corresponded to lower injury rates and associated costs (Cady, Thomas, and Karwasky, 1985). The fittest employees had only one eighth as many injuries as the least-fit employees, and unfit workers incurred twice as

many low-back injury costs as fit workers. In addition, workers' compensation claims dropped by half for the entire department in the final 8 years of the study, and disability costs declined 25%. (It should be noted that these improvements are probably the result of both the physical fitness program and changes in the administration of a return-to-work program.)

One researcher studied the effect of two 5-minute exercise breaks on musculoskeletal strain among data-entry operators. The exercises were designed to relieve cervicobrachial posture strain but also included arm, wrist, and lower-leg manipulation. In the 2 years before the introduction of the exercise program, at any one time, 7 to 12 active CTD-based workers' compensation claims were filed on behalf of injured operators. In the year following the introduction of the program, no new claims were filed. There was also an immediate 25% climb in productivity and a cost savings in less overtime reported in other areas.

Some health care professionals suggest that workers who regularly engage in vigorous, whole-body exercise such as swimming have a much lower risk for carpal tunnel syndrome and possibly other types of CTDs.

Most of the research published over the past two decades indicates that WHP reduces the incidence, severity, and associated costs of CTDs. Studies also show that regular exercisers have no greater risk of sustaining musculoskeletal injuries than nonexercisers and occasional exercisers. Nevertheless, most of the CTD-based studies focus primarily on back injuries and do not address other CTDs such as carpal tunnel syndrome and other repetitive motion injuries.

Overall, studies on the potential influence of WHP on CTDs generate several yet-unanswered questions:

1. What types of personal factors actually influence injury risk?

2. Are these factors as influential in all types of worksites or only in specific types of worksites?

3. Can specific factors be influenced by voluntary lifestyle changes resulting from a WHP intervention?

4. Which intervention makes the greatest impact for the least cost?

5. If WHP interventions carry great potential for success with CTDs, are American employers prepared to implement them?

## Strategies for CTD Prevention

Strategies recommended to employers for reducing the risk of CTDs at the workplace include adjusting workstations to fit individual needs (see figure 6.2), providing indirect light to minimize glare, providing adjustable chairs with armrests and good low-back support, supplying monitor screens, and supplying resting pads for hands and wrists. These basic strategies can be expensive but are relatively easy to implement and will significantly reduce CTDs. Strategies that are less easy to initiate—because they involve more than just purchasing new equipment—but which are less expensive and could prove just as beneficial

in the long run involve conducting education and training sessions, encouraging employees to take more breaks, and monitoring employees to make sure their work practices are not predisposing them for CTDs.

# EMPLOYEE ASSISTANCE PROGRAMS

Considering the stresses of balancing home and work life demands, quality of work life initiatives are making inroads at the workplace. According to several surveys, more employers are recognizing that employees need flexible human resource and benefit programs to help them deal with various health-related changes throughout their working years. For example, more employers are offering life cycle benefits programs that include health promotion and fitness incentives for employees and dependents. These benefit programs allow employees to tailor their benefits package according to whatever their greatest needs are at the time. Employees can choose from a varied menu of benefit offerings, including those listed in table 6.1.

Many life cycle benefits programs have evolved from employee assistance programs, or EAPs. Currently, more than 10,000 U.S. employers provide EAPs, compared to only 50 in the early 1970s. Although the original EAPs—established in the early 1950s—were designed primarily to help alcoholic workers and dependents, most of today's EAPs provide a full spectrum of services including financial counseling, substance abuse treatment, eldercare and child care assistance, and retirement planning. The most common problems addressed by today's EAPs are tied to emotional, job-related, and personal relationship problems (see figure 6.3).

Developing and operating effective life cycle benefits and EAP programs involves various administrative issues. Among the most influential issues are administrative positioning, staffing, services, sites, and participation criteria.

Integrating an EAP within a comprehensive health promotion framework is becoming more popular because doing so

- maximizes resources, especially for smaller companies with limited finances;
- makes the working environment healthier as more staff members work toward a common goal;

**Table 6.1 Components in a Life Cycle Benefits Program**

| Covered expense | You will be reimbursed for | Annual maximum |
|---|---|---|
| Healthy lifestyle | Health club membership, stopping smoking, losing weight, and so on | $400 |
| Childcare, eldercare, or adoption | Services of a nonfamily childcare or eldercare provider; for an adoption referral service | $300 |
| Financial planning | Financial planning by a qualified financial planner or the purchase of a computer-based financial planning software program | $250 |
| Legal assistance | Legal assistance in connection with wills, estates, and adoption | $200 |
| Housing assistance | After 4 years of service, for the purchase of a primary residence only | $1,000 |

- reduces the stigma associated with getting personal help—as part of a comprehensive program, workers are more likely to view EAP services in the same way as other health promotion programs; and

- helps meet the total needs of high-risk workers because programs can be tailored to help individuals with psychological problems related to alcoholism or other drug abuse, eating disorders, stress, recent heart attacks, and other personal health crises.

However, potential drawbacks of an integrated approach do exist. They include the possibility that sharing resources may limit allocations and jeopardize the potential impact of an EAP; that EAP services may be underrepresented if another

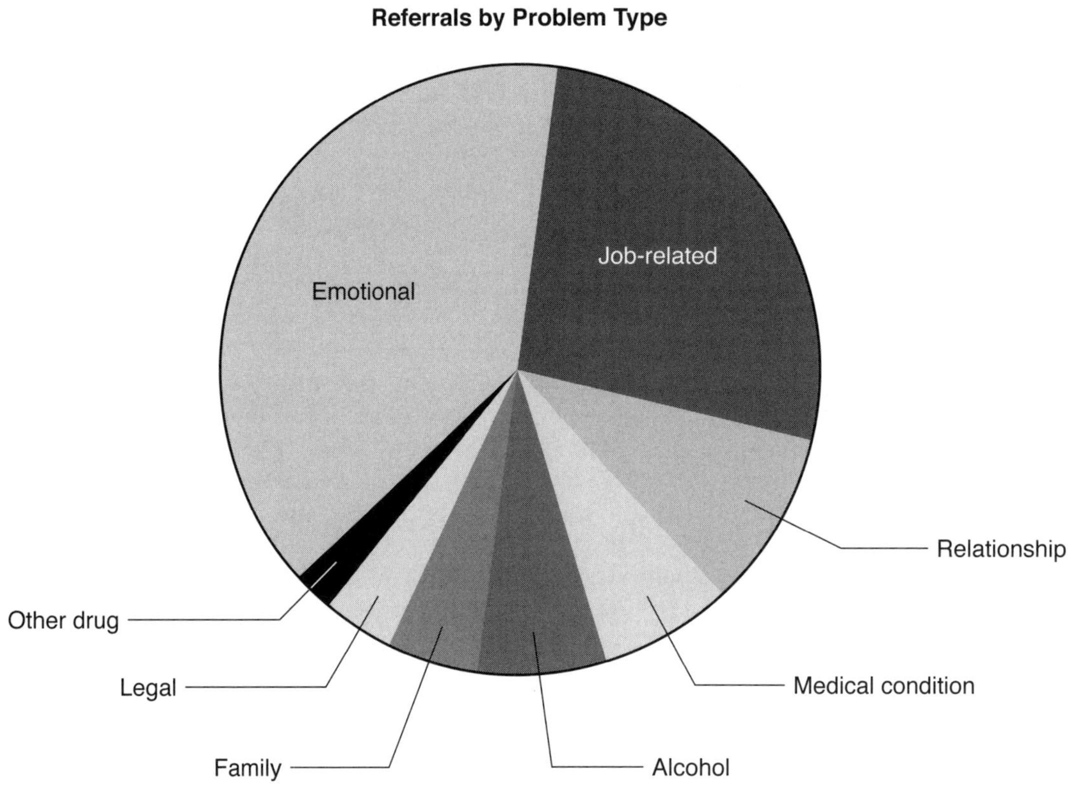

**Referrals by Problem Type**

**Figure 6.3** The most common problems reported to a randomly selected group of EAPs.

health promotion component (the fitness center, for example) becomes too visible; that employees may underestimate the importance of an EAP and not seek help; and that other health promotion programs may inadvertently try to address EAP-related issues. It is important that other programs complement EAP services rather than try to replace them.

Not just anyone should volunteer to be a member of the EAP staff. Because of the complex issues involved in dealing with the problems typically referred to EAP personnel, staffing guidelines should be followed as closely as possible. First of all, staff members should be professionally trained and certified in the areas of mental health and substance abuse.

Each staff member should be evaluated once a year. Managers and union representatives should be kept informed of any EAP staffing changes and how these changes affect responsibilities. To minimize the chance of malpractice and liability claims, employers should conduct a legal review of the EAP and keep thorough files of all EAP activity. Finally, an outside firm should evaluate the overall impact of the program every 2 to 4 years to ensure that operating standards are properly followed and designated goals are achieved.

## Establishing an EAP Site

Each on-site and off-site EAP has its own advantages and drawbacks. An on-site EAP may give a company greater opportunity to perform quality control measures, but workers may wonder whether their identities can be protected if others are aware of their EAP usage. In contrast, some workers may find it inconvenient or indiscreet to visit an off-site EAP. Whether an on-site or off-site EAP would suit your situation better may also depend on financial considerations. Larger employers are usually more likely to staff and fund an in-house EAP. However, many companies of all sizes have opted to use an alternative arrangement such as an off-site consortium or an internal referral system.

In a typical consortium arrangement, a group of employers pays a local EAP organization—for example, a local mental health center—to provide specific services to employees and dependents. Usually the fee for these services depends on the size of a workforce. For example, if an employer has a workforce of 100 employees, the employer may pay $5 for each employee ($500) plus a base rate of $1,000, for a total cost of $1,500 a year. Employers with a larger group of employees may pay the same per-employee rate of $5 but a much higher base rate.

In an internal referral arrangement, supervisors trained in EAP issues identify employees with personal problems that may be affecting their attendance, productivity, or morale. The troubled employees may be referred to an on-site EAP coordinator or to a designated EAP provider in the community for counseling. A common referral process is shown in figure 6.4. In the early 1980s, Union Pacific Railroad introduced Operation Red Block, one of the first programs in the industry to advocate peer-to-peer intervention to reduce alcohol and other drug use. (The program is named for the signal that stops traffic at railroad crossings.) If employees either refer themselves or are referred by a peer for treatment, they are exempt from the company's disciplinary process for drug use if they cooperate with their treatment plans. However, a second episode results in termination; individuals may return to work after successful treatment. Operation Red Block works in tandem with a very active EAP in which treatment plans are tailored to the needs of each individual, provided at no cost, and are confidential. This coordinated effort is responsible for the program's low recidivism rate of less than 10%.

## Substance Abuse Prevention and Treatment

A common goal of life cycle and EAP programs is to prevent and treat substance abuse. Historically, substance abuse prevention and treatment strategies centered on alcohol, but today prescription medication abuse and illegal drug use are also emphasized.

Substance abuse has a formidable economic impact on businesses. Consider these statistics:

- Lost productivity and quality defects related to substance abuse cost businesses worldwide several hundred billion dollars each year.
- Each substance abuser costs his or her employer over $7,500 a year in lost productivity, increased medical care, and damaged property.
- At least 10% of health care cost is because of substance abuse.

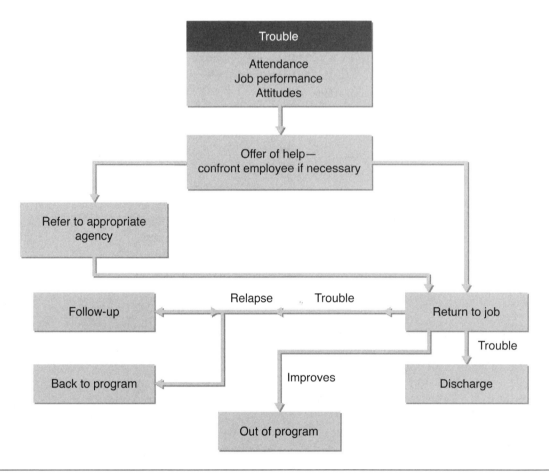

**Figure 6.4** An internal referral EAP framework.

- Approximately 10% of workers abuse alcohol or other drugs.
- Nearly 50% of all industrial accidents involve alcohol.
- Forty percent of all worksite deaths can be traced to alcohol abuse.

The National Institute of Drug Abuse (NIDA) estimates the incidence of illegal drug and heavy alcohol use among workers in specific industries as shown in table 6.2.

Following are some strategies for employers to use in dealing with substance abuse:

- Publicize a written statement on the costs and health risks associated with substance abuse and other problems covered by the EAP. The chief executive and union representatives should sign this document when appropriate. The statement should reflect management and labor philosophies and agreements that coincide with EAP objectives.
- Develop written guidelines that specify how records will be maintained; for how long; who

will have access to them; what information will be released to whom and under what conditions; and what use, if any, can be made of records for purposes of research, evaluation, and reports.

**Table 6.2 Percentage of Workers by Industry Who Use Illegal Drugs or Drink Heavily**

| Industry | PERCENTAGE OF WORKERS | |
| | Use illegal drugs | Drink heavily |
| --- | --- | --- |
| Construction | 21.6 | 17.0 |
| Repair services | 18.5 | 6.5 |
| Wholesale trade | 15.9 | 2.3 |
| Professional | 11.3 | 2.9 |
| Retail trade | 11.2 | 10.1 |
| Manufacturing | 10.3 | 3.3 |
| Finance | 9.3 | 3.8 |

• Establish written procedures to inform employees on what actions management and union representatives will take at each phase of the program.

• Operate the EAP within the standards and practices established by one or more of the following associations:

1. Employee Assistance Professional's Association (EAPA)
2. Employee Assistance Society of North America (EASNA)
3. National Institute on Alcohol Abuse and Alcoholism (NIAAA)
4. National Council on Alcoholism and Drug Dependence, Inc. (NCADD)

When a company decides to drug-test, it is wise to include goals that clearly specify provisions for ensuring the protection of an employee's identity and that all facets of the program are preserved at all times. Sound ethical procedures need to be established to protect employees' rights and minimize litigation. For example, you should hire laboratories certified by the College of American Pathologists, the National Institute of American Pathologists, or the National Institute on Drug Abuse to do the testing. To maximize accuracy, if a urine sample tests positive for drug use, the sample should then undergo either radioimmunoassay, gas chromatography, or, preferably, GC/mass spectrometry. These advanced tests (which cost between $30 and $50) break drugs into single molecules and thus confirm or contradict the presence of even small amounts of a particular drug.

Among various factors that may predispose an individual toward alcohol or other substance abuse, daily stressors can often compound other risk factors and increase a person's risk toward this unhealthy behavior.

## STRESS MANAGEMENT

According to many employee-based surveys, on-the-job stress is the most common risk factor in today's worksites. Yet, less than one of every five worksites provide employee stress management programs. These programs are in great need considering the following:

• One of four employees view their jobs as the greatest stressor in their lives.

## Recovery Rates for Substance Abusers

Recovery rates for substance abusers entering treatment through worksite interventions are the highest of any referral source; approximately 60% to 80% are successfully rehabilitated. Many companies using the most advanced techniques to identify, counsel, and treat troubled individuals are reporting favorable results from their EAP investments. One public health journal cites the following examples:

• **Allis-Chalmers:** Absenteeism dropped from 8% to 3% and the discharge rate from 95% to 8% (among participants), producing an estimated savings of over $100,000.

• **Consolidated Edison:** Nearly 60% of EAP patients are rehabilitated, and absenteeism dropped from 14 days to 4 days per year per patient.

• **Detroit Edison:** Absenteeism tied to substance abuse dropped 75%.

• **DuPont.** Approximately 66% of employees with alcoholism have been successfully rehabilitated.

• **Firestone Tire & Rubber:** Accident and sickness costs tied to substance abuse dropped 65%.

• **General Motors:** Lost work time tied to substance abuse dropped by 40%, sickness and accident claim costs associated with substance abuse dropped by 60%, and grievance proceedings tied to substance abuse dropped 50%.

• **Illinois Bell:** On-the-job disabling injuries tied to substance abuse declined 81%.

• **3M Company:** Nearly 80% of employees with alcoholism either recovered or their conditions were controlled to the point where noticeable improvements in attendance, productivity, and family and community relationships were evident.

• **McDonnell Douglas:** An estimated $5.1 million in savings (fewer health care claims and lower absenteeism) was tied to a drop in substance abuse over a 3-year period.

- Eight of 10 employees feel stress on the job, and half of them express a need for help in managing their stress.
- Four of 10 employees say their job is "very" or "extremely" stressful.
- Nearly one of three employees feel "quite a bit" or "extremely" stressed at work.
- One of four employees say they are "often" or "very often" burned out or stressed by their work.

Some industry insiders contend that U.S. workers have more stress than their European counterparts because of longer working hours and less vacation time. However, the work culture and vacation allotment in Europe is starting to mimic American patterns. Stress-related disorders at the workplace continue to increase in Japan, forcing employers to address this problem. For example, a report on Japanese companies shows the following:

- Nearly 86% of companies replied that "depression" is the most frequent disorder.
- In nearly 70% of the companies, some workers took more than a month's leave of absence from work because of an "emotional disorder." The majority of companies are working to address mental health through a "health and safety committee."

Why is worksite stress a problem for employees and employers? Distressed employees have higher rates of absenteeism, accidents, illnesses, and productivity errors than their less stressed counterparts. They also file the majority of stress-related workers' compensation claims, which have climbed to an all-time high in recent years.

More worksites are moving away from a strong emphasis on controlling symptoms of stress. Instead, they realize the value of helping people to identify the origin of stress and understand the relationship between daily stress and the development of illness and pain.

Many employers have responded by integrating stress-management counseling services within their EAPs. Additional ways to monitor and reduce employee stress include reviewing health care claims data to determine whether stress is, in fact, a problem at the worksite (e.g., monitoring medical claims, especially those classified as "mental" and "ill-defined;" converting an unused employee lounge into a quiet, dimly lighted room where employees can relax; printing monthly newsletter articles on how to identify and manage various kinds of stress; establishing a "humor room" or playing comedy videotapes for employees to view during lunch and break times; and replacing the traditional stress management program label with one that is more a more relevant to individual needs (table 6.3).

### Table 6.3 Positive Program Labels for Specific Needs

| Issue | Title |
| --- | --- |
| Expecting a baby | New Beginnings |
| Parenting | Positive Directions |
| Eldercare | Giving and Receiving |
| Time management | Taking Charge of Your Life |
| Helplessness | Asserting Yourself |
| Depression | Getting a New Perspective |

## WHAT WOULD YOU DO?

Suppose you have recently been hired by a midsize data processing company. Despite the worksite's clean exterior and neat appearance, your environmental assessment reveals that the work environment is very unhealthy because of wide-scale smoking, vending machines filled with junk food, and cramped work areas.

Your supervisor asks you to recommend specific changes to improve the work environment. Considering that you are the newest (and probably youngest) employee, which of the three challenges would you tackle first? Why? Describe your step-by-step process along with your justification.

# Promoting and Launching Worksite Programs

After reading this chapter you will be able to

→ List the four Ps of the marketing mix, and give examples of each one.

→ Identify at least six characteristics of successful WHP programs.

→ Explain the advantage of using newer cholesterol screening protocols instead of focusing only on total cholesterol.

→ Describe the difference between intrinsic and extrinsic rewards and when to use each one.

Some of the most successful WHP programs do not have expensive facilities, a large staff, or a hefty budget. However, an ingredient that most of these programs do share is a program director who is committed to identifying needs, coordinating responsibilities, and applying resources toward achieving reasonable, well-defined goals. The checklist on page 94 includes a dozen features you will typically find in successful WHP programs. Program planners may wish to copy and use the checklist to see how well their programs meet the criteria.

Developing a program that includes all 12 of these features requires careful planning before implementing the program along with regular maintenance once the program is under way.

Worksites vary tremendously, so no guarantees exist, but if a WHP program director can check at least 10 of the 12 items on the checklist, he or she can rest assured that it is positioned to be a quality program that should win popularity among participants. If the director checks fewer than 10 of the items, the program may need to be modified in ways that help the program better resemble those programs that have proven themselves to be successful.

If a program contains 10 or more of the dozen features, it is probably ready to be implemented at the worksite. Here are important tips for program directors to keep in mind while promoting WHP programs:

• When possible, offer programs on or near normal working hours and on days and times preferred by employees.

• Make program facilities available to workers on all shifts.

• When advertising the program, use a positive and catchy title for it. For instance, instead of referring to a nutrition program as "Weight Loss Program," consider using "Eating to Energize Your Life" or "Eating for the Good Life." Other examples include "Taking Charge!" (exercise program), "Smooth Transitions" (stress-management program), and "Kicking Butts" (smoking cessation program).

• Use personal testimonies from past and current participants to highlight the benefits of a specific program. To be the most inspirational, testimonies should be short and to the point.

## Checklist for a Successful Program

Choose the items that are true for your program. If you check fewer than 10, you may have more work to do.

_____ 1. Top management supports the program.

_____ 2. The company has a designated budget for health promotion.

_____ 3. The program is free or inexpensive to employees.

_____ 4. Qualified personnel operate the program.

_____ 5. The program staff seeks regular input from both management and employees.

_____ 6. Opportunities to participate in the program are convenient for all employees.

_____ 7. Health screenings and staff surveys are conducted regularly to assess employees' needs and interests.

_____ 8. Attractive and informative program materials are available for employees to use at work and at home.

_____ 9. When possible, health promotion activities are open to dependents and retirees.

_____ 10. The company's mission statement cites a healthy workforce among its top priorities.

_____ 11. The program provides both general and customized health promotion activities for employees at all work locations.

_____ 12. The company gets involved in local health promotion programs to show its commitment to improving the community's health status.

---

• Consider charging participants a small fee (e.g., $5) that can be pooled into a reward bank to purchase awards for employees who reach their personal goals.

• Explore the feasibility of providing employees with at least 1 hour of paid release time each week to participate in on-site health programs.

• Consider offering small group (interdepartmental) competitions to boost motivation and fun for participants.

• Consider offering a portion of the company's health care cost savings to employees who participate regularly in WHP programs.

Although health promotion has its own rewards, sometimes these rewards take too long for the impatient beginner. For instance, many newcomers in fitness programs quit before they have invested enough time to accrue any exercise-related benefits. Understanding this, program directors usually offer external, tangible rewards to those with consistent participation, especially in the first few weeks or months of the program. After that, external rewards may be less necessary; participants begin to enjoy the more intrinsic rewards of feeling better, increased energy, reduced stress, and an enhanced quality of life.

Early in the program, staff members need to decide what kind of external rewards work best.

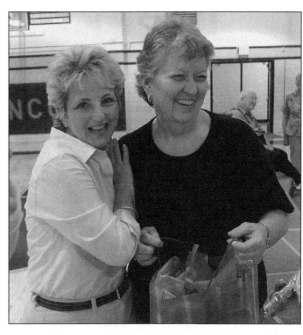

Are employees more likely to show up for a free T-shirt or hat, or would they prefer coupons to a health club or restaurant?

This information can be learned from trial and error, of course, but a simpler way to identify popular incentives is to use an incentive survey to ask employees what they prefer (see chapter 2).

Again, nothing promotes a program better than demonstrated benefits in areas that employees care about. If a weight management program helps workers lose weight and improve self-esteem, chances are good they will return for as long as the program provides these benefits. On the other hand, if employees do not see the benefits they are gaining in the program, they will need external incentives for adherence until important intrinsic benefits are more clearly seen and felt.

Plans for launching the program include (1) developing a strategy to make the program enticing to employees—that is, a marketing strategy, (2) preparing employees for action, (3) developing a health fair, (4) conducting employee health screening, (5) risk and liability management, (6) giving the program a trial run, (7) selecting rewards, and (8) coming up with ideas for maintaining participation in the program once it is up and running.

# DEVELOPING A MARKETING STRATEGY

*Marketing* is defined as an aggregate of functions involved in moving goods from producer to consumer. Depending on the goods involved, these functions might include describing the product to those who have never heard of it; explaining what the product is and how to use it; advertising the product so that consumers know it exists; monitoring the product at the developmental site to check for consistent quality; distributing the product in various quantities to match the needs of different consumer segments; transporting the product to places where the consumer can easily get to it; again monitoring the product at the distributor, wholesaler, or retailer to ensure consistent quality; and seeking feedback about the product from the consumer to learn ways to improve the product's future marketability. When people talk about "goods," we tend to think of tangible items, but the marketing principles that apply to tangibles also apply to intangibles such as WHP. As the product's "producer," the program director's job is to make the product (WHP) available and appealing to the "consumer."

Organizations with successful WHP programs usually focus their marketing efforts on the four Ps—Product, Price, Placement, and Promotion—also called the *marketing mix*.

## Product

When your product is health promotion—helping people to feel better, reduce health risks, and be more productive—you might think the product would sell itself, but unfortunately this is not the case. As with all other products or services, a health promotion program must be marketed in such a way that consumers find it attractive and worth experiencing. As summarized in table 7.1, important questions to ask about the program include, What is our service? Is it tangible, visible, and measurable? and What is the need for this service? Employees need to know precisely what they are being offered. Does the WHP program require a commitment of an hour a day or only an hour a week? Does the program offer customized options for personalized services or a "one size fits all" approach? How much flexibility is allowed for employees with busy schedules outside of work? Can employees participate during scheduled work hours? What exactly can they gain by participating in a program that promotes health? Will the benefits be financial, tangible, practical, or otherwise directly applicable to their current situation, or will they be more abstract and hard to measure? These questions and possibly others must be answered to employees' satisfaction if they are going to be enticed to try the program.

## Price

No matter how the program's expenses are covered—100% by the employer, 100% by the employee, or somewhere in between—employees must perceive that the benefits of the program outweigh their own personal costs, or they will not participate. Even if a program is free of charge in terms of money, some employees may find it too expensive in terms of time, location, special clothing, or equipment. Whether the costs are in dollars, hours, or ounces of sweat, the employees' perception must be that they have more to gain than they have to lose.

Price considerations exist from the employer's perspective as well. Some employers will find that a program is not financially feasible unless it is funded in part by the participants or participation occurs only on employees' time. Will this compromise employee participation? Will employees resent paying even a small percentage and consequently choose not to participate? Such questions need answers before the program is launched.

## Placement

Another consideration for WHP program directors and their employers is which employees to

**Table 7.1   The Four Ps of Marketing**

| Questions to address | Considerations |
|---|---|
| **PRODUCT** | |
| 1. What is our product or service?<br><br>2. Is it tangible, visible, and measurable?<br><br>3. What is the employee's (or client's) need for the product or service<br>    to look better?<br>    to feel better?<br>    to be more productive?<br>    to lower health risk?<br>    to socialize with others? | Define the product or service in precise terms. |
| **PRICE** | |
| 1. Should we charge participants?<br><br>2. Can the employee/company reasonably afford the product/service?<br><br>3. Does the product or service produce a greater benefit than cost? | Cost may be an extremely important factor in small businesses and other organizations with tight budgets. Thus, variably priced options of the product or service may be necessary. Determine the probable cost savings of the product or service. (See chapter 6 for an overview of benefit-cost analysis.) |
| **PLACEMENT** | |
| 1. Who will receive the product or service<br>    all employees?<br>    high-risk employees?<br>    only men or only women?<br><br>2. Which employees are likely to benefit from the product or service? | Consider breaking the workforce into segments based on specific attributes:<br><br>• Age<br>• Gender<br>• Family size<br>• Type of work<br>• Education level<br>• Division or department<br>• Past participation status<br>• Work shift<br>• HRA respondents<br>• Commuting time to/from work |
| **PROMOTION** | |
| 1. What types of incentives can be used to make the product or service appealing? | A demonstrated benefit must be shown for consumers to use the product or service. Use tangible incentives to create a unique selling point. Some examples include:<br><br>• Freebies (T-shirts, on-site child care, health screenings)<br>• Discounts (health insurance discount, health club membership, and so on)<br>• Personal coaching, training, or counseling |
| 2. What is the best time to promote the product or service? | Periods of layoffs, sluggish business, or merger talks may preoccupy or compel some employees to work overtime and, thus, not respond to a product or service promotion. |
| 3. Where should promotional efforts be directed? | Options include on-site (employee workstations, time clocks, cafeteria, medical clinic, safety meetings, break areas) and off-site (employees' homes). |
| 4. What promotional techniques should be used? | Options include e-mail, company Web page, newsletters, paycheck stuffers, voice mail, bulletin boards, business television channel, benefits updates, and direct mailings to employees' homes. |

focus on when starting the program. Should the program target all employees equally, or should only particular groups be targeted? Keep in mind that success or failure is often determined in the early stages of any endeavor. If the program is to receive a trial run, it might be best to include only some employees rather than all. This way, if the trial fails, the program can be adjusted and restarted without losing credibility with all employees. If all employees are targeted and the first run of the program fails, it will be more difficult to create enthusiasm again.

Some WHP programs (e.g., disease management and case management) aim at only high-risk employees because the program services are designed to meet specific needs. However, it is also true that some high-risk employees are less likely to participate in a WHP program than moderate-risk or low-risk employees are. Why is this? Part of the reason is explained in the preceding section: some workers simply feel that their cost in time or exertion is not worth the benefits they may receive from the program. The same factors that have led to their high-risk status make them less likely to sacrifice time and effort for health improvements. Conversely, employees whose healthier lifestyles keep them at relatively low risk are usually more likely to participate in a WHP program because the program is aligned with their current values. Such considerations, although potentially disheartening for program directors, need to be acknowledged and dealt with if the program is to have realistic goals and successfully counter potential pitfalls.

It can be worthwhile to vary aspects of a WHP program for different groups of employees. If possible, an employer might consider offering a cafeteria-style program in which employees choose portions of the program that they perceive best suits them. For instance, instead of focusing on nutrition or stress management for all employees in a given week, a program might give employees the option to forgo that week's emphasis and spend an additional week in a walking program instead.

Sometimes it can be advantageous to place employees into groups based on age, gender, type of work, or other factors. This allows individuals to focus on the areas they are most concerned about. For example, a group of 20- to 25-year-olds might require less aerobic training than a group of 35- to 45-year-olds, whereas the latter group might have a stronger interest in medical self-care than the former group.

## Promotion

It is important that appropriate tools be used to effectively reach as many employees as possible. In a single worksite where all employees work in a common setting, promotional displays in heavily-traveled areas may be sufficient to reach most employees (see figure 7.1). However, in worksites where employees work in different buildings, point-of-contact tools such as e-mail, paycheck stuffers, company Web site postings, and weekly safety meetings are generally used to reach disparate groups of employees.

# USING E-HEALTH TECHNOLOGY

Today, more people are turning to the Internet for health information. According to a nationwide randomized telephone survey of adults, of the hundreds of millions of people who daily surf the Internet, more than 60% use the resource for personal health information (Landro, 2005). This number is expected to increase as much as 5% a year in this population, commonly referred to as "cyberchondriacs" by pollsters. With the advent of the Internet and related communication options that continuously appear in our daily lives, many WHP professionals are using these new technologies in various educational and informational functions. This evolving phenomenon can be classified as *e-health technology* and defined as the application of Internet and other related technologies to improve the access, efficiency, effectiveness, and quality of clinical and business practices used by organizations, practitioners, and consumers to improve and maintain the health status of individuals and organizations.

Many worksites have on-site access to Internet and related technologies for employees to use in various WHP activities. In particular, numerous worksites have expanded their e-health technological capabilities beyond the Internet by building their own intranet system comprised of integrated company-specific databases. An intranet system essentially gives employees one-stop access to different types of information and resources from various departments. In many companies, employees can use this integrated system to quickly inquire about WHP program schedules, log in exercise points, trace their readiness-to-change progress, learn new stress management techniques, access a smoking cessation hotline, and acquire a host of other self-help news

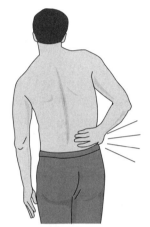

**Health Committee Members:** ——— Promotion

**Please Post on all Bulletin Boards**

——— Product

# GET BACK TO HEALTH

**Are you tired of sore back muscles and back aches?**
**Want more energy for life?**
**Then, it's time to get back to health!**

Placement ———

**For anyone concerned about their back**

Price ——— Free! ——— Unique selling point

All participants receive a free back screening

**Monday, November 25th**
**Conference Room #14**
**4:30–5:30 PM**

✂ - - - - - - - - - - - - - - - - - - - - - - - - - - - - - -

**Sign-Up Form**

Name ————————————— Dept. ——————

Reason for attending program
_____

Please return form to Health & Safety Office
by November 1st. *Thank you!*

Figure 7.1  A sample low-back program promotion poster highlighting the four Ps of the marketing mix.
Reprinted, by permission, from Robert E. Mason Company.

bits and resources. Commercial vendors are also offering these programs, which typically include a virtual fitness center, nurse line, disease management services, and an e-health Web site.

Health promotion professionals can use e-health management tools to effectively launch and implement WHP programs, events, and activities in a timely and cost-effective manner. However, in doing so, they need to use some time-tested techniques to maximize the impact of their e-health efforts. First, take the time to get in-house communications experts involved in your marketing plan and related goal-setting initiatives. It is also important to provide regular updates to senior managers to secure their continued support for the program by helping them to see how e-health management resources relate to the company's goals and financial health. Although communication tools vary from worksite to worksite, a few communication channels appear to work well in most organizations, such as the following:

- Broadcast e-mail messaging
- Internet mailings
- Home mailings
- Intranet feature postings
- Announcements during company meetings, events, and activities
- Promotional posters and table tents in highly visible locations at the worksite

Second, it takes an integrated multidisciplinary team to implement and maintain a highly successful e-health initiative. The most successful e-health initiatives are led by a key individual who takes on the sole responsibility of coordinating and delegating with all of the necessary players. A common approach is to form teams made up of diverse departments including communications, risk management, benefits, human resources, health and safety, information services, and any other human capital interest groups. In organizations with multisite operations, it is important to establish a key contact at each location to spearhead and coordinate these functions. Third, it is important to realize that e-health management is a platform, not a program. According to industry experts, if e-health is to be fully optimized, organizations need to recognize this approach as a company-wide, Web-based platform that addresses human capital, and not simply the next health improvement program. Fourth, in building an integrated e-health platform, it is necessary to take inventory of your company's employee health resources (departments, events, programs, and incentives). Once these resources are identified, establishing the integrative opportunities is more evident for decision makers. Finally, it is essential to position e-health to reach as many people in as many ways as possible. Before any of the preceding four principles can be institutionalized, the overall infrastructure must be seen as moving—or, better yet, transforming—the organization's culture in a new and positive direction. Perhaps the most relevant example is the ability of an e-health platform to synchronize with the newest business trend of electronic self-service. This feature is designed to save money and time by eliminating administrative tasks and includes venues such as online health benefits enrollment, online financial planning, and office procurement.

## PREPARING EMPLOYEES TO TAKE ACTION

In realizing how difficult it is to motivate employees to participate in WHP programs on a consistent basis, many worksite health and fitness professionals have incorporated the stages of change (readiness to act) model in their programming efforts. James Prochaska, PhD, and Carlo DiClemente, PhD, created this model to describe the various levels of a person's readiness or motivation to act (Proschaska, Norcross, and DiClemente, 1994). It is comprised of the following five stages:

1. *Precontemplation*: The person has not considered doing any health-enhancement action.
2. *Contemplation*: The person is considering action but has not yet acted.
3. *Preparation*: The person has intentions to act soon and is planning a course of action.
4. *Action*: The person is actively participating.
5. *Maintenance*: The person has been participating for at least 6 months and has been working to prevent a relapse.

Because the bulk of your WHP marketing efforts may focus on persons in stages 1, 2, and 3, it is important to structure your resources around all employees, including those in stages 4 and 5.

Far too often, WHP staff members assume that persons in the action and maintenance stages will automatically continue to be loyal participants in their programs, only to be surprised when these "diehards" end up on the sidelines because of an injury, work-related changes, greater family demands, boredom, or other unforeseen circumstances that take them out of action.

In realizing the need to tailor their motivational efforts around the diverse needs and interests of employees, many WHP providers are using high-tech and low-tech strategies to reach more workers. In our high-tech society, one of the fastest-growing motivational strategies health and fitness professionals use is actually a low-tech phenomenon called coaching.

What is coaching? The International Coach Federation (ICF) defines *coaching* as an ongoing professional relationship that helps people produce extraordinary results in their lives, careers, businesses, or organization. Through the process of coaching, clients deepen their learning, improve their performance, and enhance their quality of life. Coaching accelerates the client's progress by providing greater focus and awareness of choice. The interaction creates clarity and moves the client into action. Major features of health coaching include all of the following:

• *Health assessment*: A health risk appraisal or health screening is used to establish a baseline on the client

• *Assessment data review*: A process during which the coach uses the data to establish an outline of procedures to use in guiding the initial session(s) with the client; the coach may or may not share the outline with the client

• *Initial coaching session*: A session in which the coach and client discuss and assess the client's readiness to act and ways to proceed

• *Follow-up coaching sessions*: Regularly scheduled sessions held to assess the client's current status, recent progress, and ways to continuously improve

Table 7.2 describes various coaching strategies that can be integrated into and complement WHP programs.

## Program Adherence

Once a program has been successfully promoted and is under way, program planners need strategies for motivating employees to stick with the program. Many employees are excited at the beginning but lose interest if they don't see immediate results for their efforts. Because perceptible changes in a person's health status and fitness level are usually gradual, it may be necessary to offer external rewards until an intrinsic reward—such as feeling better—becomes a self-perpetuating force. Following are some other suggestions for helping employees stay with a program. (Note that extrinsic rewards may be more effective if they are offered only after the initial momentum has slowed.)

• Help employees set realistic goals. Break a long-term goal into short-term goals (e.g., split a proposed 10% weight loss into six monthly goals of losing 5 pounds a month).

• Stress the need to begin slowly, especially in exercise and weight loss efforts.

• Give regular verbal support and written feedback to all participants while assessing their progress.

• Establish a point system in which participants can redeem wellness bucks for mugs, T-shirts, self-care books, and other prizes.

• Use a map to signify the distance walked, biked, or swum by participants in a coast-to-coast cross-country challenge, and give awards at certain landmarks or cities.

• Feature a participant of the month for outstanding attendance or performance.

• Sponsor a fun run and walk with participants predicting their finish times; reward those with the closest actual times.

• Use an honor system to reward employees who promote their health at home and on the road.

For example, create personal health promotion checksheets for specific topics (exercise, nutrition, weight loss, smoking cessation). Have employees check off their weekly accomplishments and submit them at regular intervals for prizes (see sample checksheet on page 102).

One of the most popular wellness incentive campaigns used at many worksites is to offer points for participation. Many program directors think it allows flexibility to the degree that each employee can select what he or she considers valuable—cash, prizes, or even time off work. When setting up a point program, some program directors stack the deck by offering fewer points for popular programs and more points for less popular but valuable programs.

**Table 7.2  Coaching Strategies Tailored to Specific Stages of Readiness**

| Stage | Coaching strategies |
|---|---|
| 1. Precontemplation | • Assess personal health status of client.<br>• Assess personal priorities with client.<br>• Assess readiness level to act.<br>• Inform client that taking action is: (1) important, (2) beneficial, and (3) achievable. |
| 2. Contemplation | • Ask open-ended questions to assess client's intentions and readiness to act.<br>• Avoid giving action-oriented instructions such as fitness classes and diet plans.<br>• Help client understand that the advantages of acting outweigh the disadvantages of not being able to live a quality lifestyle (e.g., "Acting now will help you feel better, be more productive, sleep better, reduce premature illnesses," and so on).<br>• Use reflective listening to build client's self-confidence to take action (e.g., "It seems as if you see a connection between a lack of regular exercise and being overweight, lacking energy," and so on).<br>• Help client identify positive role models that will support his or her actions.<br>• Ask client to set a personal goal that is achievable and can be incorporated into his or her current schedule without much interference. |
| 3. Preparation | • Ask client to set a goal, if he or she hasn't already done so.<br>• Help client identify an incentive to take action.<br>• Ask client to identify potential barriers to act and ways to overcome them.<br>• Encourage the client to act on his or her goal in progressive steps. |
| 4. Action | • Reinforce client's good actions.<br>• Encourage client to track personal progress and tell others.<br>• Ask client to identify potential barriers to act and ways to overcome them.<br>• Encourage client to act on his or her goal in progressive steps.<br>• In subsequent coaching sessions, encourage client to move beyond the initial goal (e.g., exercise 2 more minutes per session than before). |
| 5. Maintenance | • Reinforce client's good actions.<br>• Encourage client to review personal progress and revise goals, if necessary.<br>• Encourage client to track personal progress and tell others.<br>• Ask client to identify potential barriers to act and ways to keep them from causing a relapse.<br>• Provide client with handouts, articles, testimonies from others, and personal screening results to reinforce the benefits of maintenance.<br>• In subsequent coaching sessions, encourage client to personally set a new goal. |

One common question about incentive-based programs is, Should you pay for participation or for results? If you choose to incentivize with results, consider some regulations relevant to the Health Information Portability and Accountability Act (HIPAA). For example, group health insurance plans cannot discriminate with respect to employee eligibility or premiums, but employers may implement a bona fide wellness program, also called a disease prevention or health promotion program, without being in violation. In doing so, four major criteria comprise a bona fide program:

1. Any reward or discount cannot exceed a fixed percentage of the planned cost of the employee's health insurance coverage for the year.

2. The program must (a) be designed to promote health and prevent disease, (b) be open to employees at least once a year, and (c) enable employees to earn whatever incentives are offered within 1 year.

3. The rewards must be available to similarly situated employees. For example, you may legally allow full-time employees to participate but exclude part-time employees. You may also classify by length of service and disallow new (probationary) employees from participating. However, when it comes to something like a smoking cessation program, you must have an alternative standard of success for people who cannot comply with your behavioral objectives

## Sample Exercise-Based Checksheet

*Instructions:* Please calculate points earned for each week and the entire month. Turn the checksheet in to your supervisor by the first day of each month. Point credits are as follows:

- 15 minutes of nonstop activity = 2 points
- 20 minutes of nonstop activity = 3 points
- 25 minutes of nonstop activity = 4 points
- 30 minutes of nonstop activity = 5 points
- 35+ minutes of nonstop activity = 6 points

### Personal Health Promotion Checksheet

| Week number | TYPE OF EXERCISE COMPLETED | | | | | Total points |
| --- | --- | --- | --- | --- | --- | --- |
| | Walking | Biking | Swimming | Jogging/running | Other (list) | |
| 1 | 2 | 3 | | | | |
| | 2 | 3 | | | | |
| | 2 | 3 | | | | 15 |
| 2 | | 3 | | | | |
| | | | 3 | | | |
| | 2 | | | | | |
| | 2 | | | | | 10 |
| 3 | 3 | | | | | |
| | 3 | 2 | | | | |
| | | 4 | | | | 12 |
| 4 | 4 | 4 | | | | |
| | | 4 | | | | |
| | | 2 | | | | 10 |
| *Monthly total:* | | | | | | 47 |

because of a medical or physical condition. For example, smoking is considered an addiction and, as such, if you offer an incentive to quit smoking, you must offer an alternative standard of success so that smokers can have access to the reward on an equivalent basis.

4. Finally, the alternative standard of success must be disclosed to the same extent as the general standard of success.

Because financial incentives are believed to be one of the strongest incentives, more employers are offering financial wellness banks or health care accounts to employees who complete an annual health assessment or participate in specific WHP programs. Employees who meet specified criteria can access a personal account of company-funded dollars (generally $250 to $750 a year) to apply up front toward their medical insurance premium, deductible, or co-payment or to be reimbursed for approved medical care services.

## Attracting Nonparticipants and High-Risk Employees

While incentives and rewards work well at many worksites, all companies have their share of nonparticipants. Such "no-shows" are costly, as they often have greater health risks, which eventually lead to premature illnesses and disabilities that, in large part, are paid by their employers. For example, three large-scale studies conducted on employees at Ceridian Corporation, Steelcase Corporation, and DaimlerChrysler Corporation show that workers with potentially modifiable risk factors (e.g., smoking, obesity, and inactivity) are absent more and incur greater health care expenses than lower-risk employees. Presumably, these individuals could benefit from WHP activities, but less than 5% of all high-risk employees actually participate in WHP programs.

As more employers become aware of the strong correlation between an employee's health status and health care costs, they offer customized incentives and rewards to this hard-to-reach sector. However, to be successful, program planners first need to identify each sector's values, interests, and readiness to act.

A typical workforce may consist of four (or more) segments. The first group is often called the "diehards" because of their very strong interest and regular participation in health enhancement activities. These employees are the easiest to recruit and are often willing to assist WHP staff in various capacities (e.g., publicize WHP programs to coworkers).

The second segment of the workforce are those employees who express "an interest" in their health but often need tangible incentives and regular encouragement from family members, coworkers, and staff members to regularly participate in health enhancement activities.

A third segment, perhaps best called the "conditionals," might participate if the conditions are personally appealing, such as a free program on company time. They are also more likely to prefer participating with a buddy or in a group with their immediate coworkers.

A fourth segment, the "resisters," is the toughest group to motivate because these employees have little interest in their personal health and often delay lifestyle changes until a major crisis such as a heart attack has occurred. Unfortunately, many resisters have never had a healthy lifestyle and thus cannot appreciate the many benefits of good health.

No secret recipe exists for motivating the resisters—which doesn't mean that program planners should not continue to try to get these employees involved. To do so, however, requires more creativity and perseverance in developing, marketing, and implementing WHP programs for this challenging audience. Using interest surveys and other assessment tools (see chapter 2) can help staff members design appealing programs. The good news is, a WHP program can be successful without engaging every employee. In most cases, the success or failure of a program will depend on the extent to which customized promotional campaigns and programs can be offered in synch with employees' likes and capabilities. Essentially, carefully targeted incentives and rewards that fit individual and group preferences offer the greatest potential. In addition, whenever possible, it is best to use promotional strategies that include awareness and hands-on activities such as a health fair.

# DEVELOPING A HEALTH FAIR

One of the best ways to generate employee health awareness and program participation is a worksite health fair that includes colorful exhibits, audiovisual displays, interactive kiosks, educational materials, and various health screenings. To minimize the labor-intensive nature of planning a health fair, program planners may wish to ask suitable employees to assist them in preparing the location, setting up exhibits, and distributing promotional materials for the health fair. Finding volunteers may be easier if management allows employees to help on company time; however, many employees (the diehards) will usually be willing to volunteer under most circumstances. Consider the following organizations or individuals as possible health fair exhibitors:

- County health department
- Fire, rescue, and police departments
- Local health care facilities
- Medical, dental, and nursing personnel
- Private optometrists and chiropractors
- Certified massage therapists
- Community health associations (heart, cancer, lung, diabetes, asthma, and so on)
- College or university faculty and students in health-related disciplines

After receiving a verbal agreement from an organization or individual exhibitor, it is important to seal the commitment by following up in writing. This letter will also serve as a notice to all who participate that the health fair is a nonprofit event and that the company holding the fair will not accept responsibility for any losses or damages incurred during the fair. To avoid any possible legal problems, the company's WHP director will need to receive a signed copy of the letter from all participants. The company holding the health fair can use a modified version of the sample letter shown on page 104 to suit its circumstances.

# Sample Letter to Health Fair Exhibitors

Dear _____ :
  (Health Promotion Exhibitor/Vendor)

Thank you for expressing interest in our health fair, to be held on November 25 from 8 a.m. to 5 p.m. Participation by _____ such as _____ will help make the
  (individuals/organizations)                    (you/yours)
event huge success. This letter confirms our arrangement for your participation in our _____.
  (event name)

Your participation at the health fair (describe service such as give a presentation, present an exhibit, conduct a health screening, and so on) will be as an independent contractor of and not as an agent for or an employee of (health fair host company). *[If contractor will be doing an invasive, diagnostic, or potentially risky procedure, include the next paragraph.]*

_____ shall indemnify and hold _____ and their
  (Contractor name)                                      (health fair host company)
respective agents and employees harmless from any and all manner of loss, whatsoever (including reasonable costs of litigation and attorneys' fees) which_____ may hereafter incur,
                                                                              (health fair host company)
become responsible for, or pay out as a result of death or bodily injury to any person or destruction or damage to any property arising out of _____ negligence (or that of their respective
                                                        (health fair host company)
negligence (or that of their respective agents and employees), or in connection with the services provided by Contractor, except to the proportionate extent that such loss, liability, damage or claim was due to the willful misconduct of _____, its respective agents, and its employees.
                                  (health fair host company)

*[If the contractor will be doing an invasive, diagnostic, or potentially risky procedure or will be providing a piece of equipment on which trial uses will be offered, include the next paragraph.]*

As an independent contractor, you are responsible for having current general and professional *[include also "product" liability if the contractor is an equipment seller who is bringing in equipment which individuals will use]* liability coverage (minimum of $1,000,000). Please return copies of the appropriate certificates of insurance with this letter.

*[If the contractor is a sole proprietor or not affiliated with an established and reputable organization, such as a local hospital, and if the service is an invasive, diagnostic, or potentially risky procedure, include the following paragraph.]*

Please prepare an Informed Consent and Release of Liability form for individuals to sign before taking part in your service. _____ should be released from all liabilities associated
                              (health fair host company)
with your service. Enclose a copy of the form with your confirmation.

Your services will be provided at no charge to _____. *[If individuals desiring*
                                              (health fair host company)
*service will pay, note fee schedule.]*

We appreciate your participation in making the health fair a success. If you understand and agree to these arrangements and requirements, sign in the space provided. To participate in the health fair, the exhibitor must sign and return the original copy of this letter, along with any required documents named above by _____. If you have any questions about these requests, please call me at _____.
  (date)                                                                                          (phone number)

Sincerely,

_____ (health fair host company representative)

Acknowledged and agreed to by _____ (signature of exhibitor)

Name (please print) _____ Date _____

# Planning Framework

When planning the worksite health fair, program planners need to consider their compiled data on employee needs and interests (collected though various techniques discussed in chapter 2). This information is helpful in progressing through the three phases of building a health fair: preliminary planning, development, and implementation.

*Phase I: Preliminary Planning*

1. Determine primary health fair goals.
2. Review and rank employees' health needs using company health records (group accident data, group medical claims data, and workers' compensation data).
3. Identify and assess on-site and community health resources.
4. Develop and distribute a survey to local health promotion professionals and health care providers to determine their interest in participating in a health fair.
5. Compile survey information into a database showing names, services or products, and contact information for prospective vendors and exhibitors.

*Phase II: Health Fair Development*

1. Choose an on-site health fair coordinator.
2. Develop a theme and logo (see table 7.3 for ideas).
3. Set locations, dates, and times for the event.
4. Prepare a working budget.
5. Confirm participation details with prospective vendors and exhibitors.
6. Share the health fair layout and setup requirements with all vendors and exhibitors.
7. Design and prepare publicity materials (e.g., newsletter articles, flyers, and posters).
8. Use various media venues to encourage employee participation.

*Phase III: Program Implementation*

1. Contact and inform all vendors, exhibitors, and on-site personnel about final arrangements including setup procedures, dismantling times, and procedures.
2. Conduct a mock walk-through to check traffic flow, spacing, and supervision needs.
3. Open the Fair!

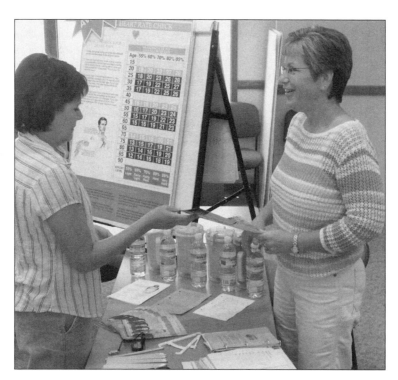

Health fairs may highlight back-health programs for workers in labor-intensive jobs, prenatal health education programs for women, exercise programs for persons who sit a lot, and consumer education and medical self-care programs for employees who frequently use health care services.

# Promotion

Organizers can use posters, bulletin boards, newsletters, e-mail, and other internal resources to advertise the health fair and subsequent events to employees. For greatest exposure, promotional materials should be displayed at key locations at least 2 weeks before the fair. Targeting promotional efforts to specific employee groups also can enhance participation. Groups can be classified by various characteristics such as age, gender, race, specific risk factors, previous participation, and so on.

Timing is obviously an important factor in promoting new programs. Numerous worksites launch their health fairs in January, in synch with employees' New Year's resolutions. Also, consider promoting specific programs around various state and national health and fitness campaigns such as the National Employee Health & Fitness Day in mid-May (see table 7.3). To encourage a good turnout with active participation, consider using Plan A or Plan B as follows:

*Plan A*

1. As they enter the health fair, give each employee a personal "health card" (e.g., large index card) with specific instructions to follow.

2. Ask them to read and follow the instructions listed on the card to qualify for a healthy reward at the health fair as well as qualify for a grand prize (to be awarded at the end of the health fair).

3. Ask each exhibitor or vendor to stamp the employee's card *after they participate* in the activity. It will deter employees from expecting they can simply appear at each station to get their card stamped.

*Plan B*

1. Have each vendor type three or four easy questions pertaining to their exhibit, and display them on a stand-up display card at their respective locations.

2. Make a quiz with "true" and "false" columns corresponding to each question. Give employees one answer sheet for each exhibit, and instruct them to write their name and department number on each answer sheet.

3. Encourage them to complete an answer sheet at each exhibit and check it for right and wrong answers that appear on the back side of the quiz. After checking all answers, employees can place it in a drop box and enter a random drawing—every 30 minutes, for example—for various prizes donated by the exhibitors.

## Table 7.3  Themes and Occasions for Promoting Health Fairs

| Program | Health fair theme | Occasions | Month |
|---------|-------------------|-----------|-------|
| Physical fitness | Physical Fitness | Physical Fitness and Sports Month | May |
| | | Family Health and Fitness Day USA | September |
| | | Women's Health and Fitness Day | September |
| Nutrition and weight control | Healthy Weights | Healthy Weight Week | January |
| | | Nutrition Month | March |
| | | 5-A-Day Month | September |
| | | Diabetes Month | November |
| | Heart Health | Heart Month | February |
| | | Women's Heart Day | February |
| | | High Blood Pressure Education Month | May |
| | | Stroke Awareness Month | May |
| Back health | Healthy Joints | Correct Posture Month | May |
| | | Arthritis Month | May |
| | | Osteoporosis Awareness and Prevention Month | May |

| Program | Health fair theme | Occasions | Month |
| --- | --- | --- | --- |
| Prenatal health | Healthy Moms, Healthy Babies | March of Dimes Walk | April |
| | | World Health Day | April |
| Smoking control | Healthy Breathing | Clean Air Month | May |
| | | Healthy Lung Month | October |
| | | Great Smoke Out | November |
| | | Lung Cancer Awareness Month | November |
| | | Asthma and Allergy Awareness Month | May |
| AIDS education and HIV disease prevention | Facts for Life | National Black HIV/AIDS Awareness Day | February |
| | | World AIDS Day | December |
| Medical self-care and health care consumerism | Cancer Prevention and Awareness | Cervical Cancer Screening Month | January |
| | | Colorectal Cancer Awareness Month | March |
| | | Cancer Control Month | April |
| | | Skin Cancer Awareness Month | May |
| | | Ovarian Cancer Awareness Month | September |
| | | Prostate Cancer Awareness Month | September |
| | | Breast Cancer Awareness Month | October |
| | | Mammography Day | October |
| | Healthy Awareness | Wise Health Consumer Month | February |
| | | Kidney Month | March |
| | | Healthy Vision Month | May |
| | | Immunization Awareness Month | August |
| | | Cholesterol Education Month | September |
| | | Liver Awareness Month | October |
| | | Talk About Prescriptions Month | October |
| | | Healthy Skin Month | November |
| | Personal Wellness | Better Sleep Month | May |
| | | Mental Health Month | May |
| | | Headache Awareness Week | June |
| | | International Massage Week | July |
| | | Men's Health Week | July |
| | | Depression Screening Day | October |
| Occupational injury | Safety | Safety Month | July |
| | | Workplace Eye Health and Safety Month | March |
| | | Drive Safely at Work Week | October |
| Employee assistance program (EAP) and quality of work life (QWL) | Substance Abuse, Child Care, Eldercare, Financial and Retirement Planning | Drunk and Drugged Driving Prevention Month | December |
| | | Child Care Awareness Days | June |
| | | Family Caregiver Week | May |
| | | Financial Awareness Week | July |
| | | National Retirement Planning Week | November |
| Stress management | Workplace Stress | National Stress Awareness Day | November |

# CONDUCTING EMPLOYEE HEALTH SCREENING

Any time employees participate in employer-sponsored health fairs and other types of WHP events, an employer assumes some degree of risk. Legally, an employer may be held liable for an employee's injury if

- an employee is injured while participating in an employer-mandated program or activity,
- the employer benefits from the employee's attendance or participation in the program he or she is injured in, or
- the employee is injured on the job.

Although WHP-related lawsuits are rare, worksites should naturally take steps to minimize any liability risk. For example, many companies have positioned their programs so that workers' compensation insurance or private liability insurance covers any program-related or on-the-job injuries. Another strategy is to develop a screening program that effectively identifies high-risk employees for appropriate referral into specific programs in tune with their capabilities and needs.

Employers that offer programs or facilities with admission or participation policies that exclude or limit certain individuals from program activities, should carefully review the requirements of Great Britain's Disability Discrimination Act (DDA) or the Americans With Disabilities Act (ADA). For example, using safety-screening criteria is probably permissible under the Act, provided the criteria are based on actual risks, not stereotypical ones. The ADA stipulates that employers cannot discriminate on the basis of a person's disability, so it is essential to know what types of conditions are considered to be legitimate disabilities. Under the ADA, an individual with a disability is a person who

- has a physical or mental impairment that substantially limits one or more major life activities,
- has a record of such an impairment, or
- is regarded as having such an impairment (ADA, 2005).

Specifically, the ADA defines a physical impairment this way:

[A]ny physiological disorder or condition, cosmetic disfigurement, or ana-tomical loss affecting one or more of the following body systems: neurological, musculoskeletal, special sense organs, respiratory (including speech organs), cardiovascular, reproductive, digestive, genitourinary, hemic and lymphatic, skin, and endocrine. (ADA, 2005)

The ADA defines a mental impairment this way:

[a]ny mental or psychological disorder, such as mental retardation, organic brain syndrome, emotional or mental illness, and specific learning disabilities.

Worksites that use a screening system to admit or exclude individuals from exercise or recreation programs may have to modify their policies to accommodate the provisions of the law and should seek legal advice for guidance in reviewing current policies. Also, health professionals responsible for developing and administering health-screening protocols should comply with the following standards:

- Screening techniques should be medically warranted and conducted only by authorized, competent professionals.
- Before employees are screened, they should be informed of the purpose of the screening and any other pertinent information.
- Post follow-up screening should be conducted in order for program personnel to interpret screening results for employees on an individualized basis.
- Screening should not rely solely on a physical exam to evaluate a person's total health status. A physical examination should identify organic signs and symptoms, such as high blood pressure or a heart murmur, but a health screen should also review lifestyle habits and family history.

Virtually all employees have some level of measurable health risk. Some studies that indicate the prevalence of multiple behavioral (lifestyle) risk factors are shown in table 7.4.

Researchers at Michigan State University conducted a study in 2005 suggesting the preceding estimates are far too optimistic. The researchers found that only 3% of the 153,000 American adults randomly sampled achieved low-risk status on all four of the targeted lifestyle characteristics (didn't smoke, had healthy body weight, ate at least five

**Table 7.4  Range of Health Risks**

| Percentage of employees (Approximate) | Number of risk factors |
|---|---|
| 10% | 0 |
| 33% | 1 |
| 41% | 2 |
| 14% | 3 |
| 3% | 4 |

servings of fruits and vegetables a day, and regularly exercised) (Reeves and Rafferty, 2005).

Because risk factors vary in type and prevalence from worksite to worksite, it is important to have screening procedures that detect risk factors in all employees who may participate in a WHP program. In particular, any selected procedure should factor in age, gender, current health status, family history, activity level, and occupation.

Traditional screening techniques may cost less than some contemporary methods; but the newer, more expensive techniques might be better at revealing problems. For example, traditional health screening focused heavily on a person's total cholesterol level when estimating an individual's heart disease risk. However, since the late 1990s, researchers have found that a person's LDL (low-density lipoprotein) level, the ratio of their total cholesterol-to-HDL cholesterol level, and their level of CRP (c-reactive protein) are more accurate, though slightly more expensive, than a person's total cholesterol level. Essentially, the extra cost of administering a more expensive screening technique is usually more than offset by the long-term savings of preventing an injury or a heart attack.

One large-scale study conducted in a major medical center determined the cost-effectiveness of various screening techniques on a population demographically similar to that of the U.S. workforce. One thousand adults were subjected to 10 different health-screening techniques to determine each method's validity (accuracy) and reliability (consistency). Overall, the five most cost-effective techniques were

1. health risk appraisal,
2. history and physical exam,
3. chem-12 (blood analysis),
4. urinalysis, and
5. CBC (complete blood count).

As cost-effective a screening tool as it may be, health risk appraisal (HRA) cannot identify all health problems and should be used in conjunction with other screenings. For example, many worksites supplement a person's health or medical history with an HRA. In all situations, only authorized personnel should distribute and maintain HRAs. Otherwise, some employees may perceive that management could use certain types of information (e.g., alcohol intake, cigarette smoking, and current health problems) as a basis for discrimination or dismissal.

## Preexercise Screening

In many worksites, on-site fitness screenings are conducted on employees to determine their health status, fitness level, and exercise capabilities. Unfortunately, some employees fail to show up for this important screening, which is often time-consuming and labor-intensive. One way to minimize no-shows is to first ask employees to complete an appropriate questionnaire, omitting the biomedical section (blood pressure, cholesterol, blood glucose, and so on). Screening personnel then review the questionnaires to identify employees who are not high risk and permit them to enter the program. After participating in several sessions, employees are called in individually for their personal biomedical measurement. Employees failing to attend a minimum number of exercise sessions do not receive the biomedical screening until they do so and, likewise, are not permitted to exercise in the program.

Before employees enter an exercise, fitness, or recreational program, they should be physically screened and cleared for participation. A preexercise screening protocol based on an employee's age and known risk factors is illustrated in figure 7.2.

Diagnostic laboratory testing is indicated if CHD risk factors include hyperlipidemia (high blood fats), hyperglycemia (high blood sugar), or hyperuricemia (blood in urine).

In developing a preexercise screening protocol, health professionals should remember that exercise stress testing in a symptom-free population may detect more false positives than true positives. A false positive means that the test result indicates that something is wrong when in fact nothing is wrong. Moreover, an exercise ECG has limited value in detecting or predicting coronary artery disease in asymptomatic persons with no known risk factors.

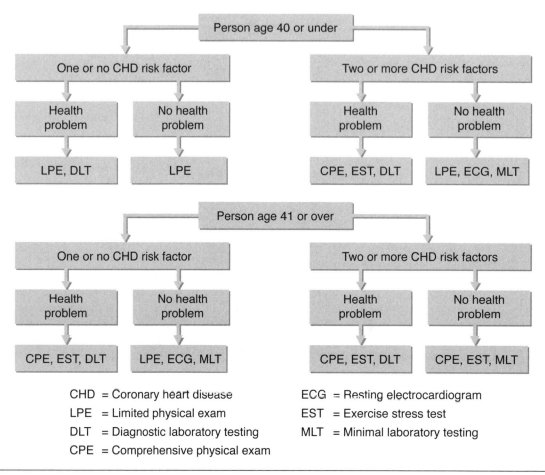

**Figure 7.2** A sample preexercise screening protocol.

Two types of preexercise tests exist: (1) symptom-limited, ECG-monitored, graded exercise tests (GXTs) and (2) submaximal tests.

GXTs should be conducted in a clinical setting, by trained personnel, and under a physician's direct supervision. The GXT protocol, administered to the subject on a motorized treadmill, is specifically designed to detect coronary ischemia (when the heart muscle receives inadequate oxygen because of diseased or blocked coronary arteries), and to determine functional capacity and safety of exercise for at-risk and symptomatic persons. Individuals at such risk and in need of the GXT protocol include persons who exhibit one or more of the following risk factors:

- Cigarette smoking
- Diabetes mellitus
- Family history of high blood cholesterol or heart disease
- Obesity

- High blood pressure (systolic over 160, diastolic over 90)
- Other high-risk condition as defined by a physician

Submaximal testing is used to determine an employee's fitness level and to assist in prescribing the right type and amount of exercise. A submaximal test can be administered with a bicycle ergometer, which is considerably less expensive than a motorized treadmill. To determine the appropriate testing protocol for each employee, it is essential to follow screening guidelines established by the American College of Sports Medicine (ACSM) or the American Heart Association (AHA). In all cases, the selected protocol should be scientifically based and tailored to each individual's overall health status. For example, a common approach is to group employees into the following classes for preexercise screening purposes:

- Class I—Healthy, conditioned individuals of all ages

- Class II—Healthy, inactive individuals under age 35
- Class III—Healthy, inactive individuals over age 35
- Class IV—Conditioned individuals of all ages with major coronary risk factors, cardiovascular disease, or both
- Class V—Inactive individuals of all ages with major coronary risk factors
- Class VI—Inactive individuals of all ages with either acute or chronic cardiovascular disease
- Class VII—Individuals for whom exercise is contraindicated

Employees in classes I, II, or III should have the submaximal test. Those in all other classes should have the symptom-limited GXT. Employees in class VII may not be tested at all.

## Other Risk and Liability Management Strategies

Employers are ultimately responsible for the safety of their WHP programs and must minimize the prospect of participants' injuries. Before they enter any type of employer-sponsored exercise program, employees should be informed in writing of their personal responsibility in meeting all preexercise clearance requirements. Most companies require employees to complete an informed consent form before participating. However, for maximum protection, employers should develop clear and concise policies requiring each participant to read such releases in the presence of a staff member and to acknowledge his or her understanding in writing. Without such documentation, an employee may claim that he or she signed the release unwittingly. It is a good idea to consult legal counsel in developing and reviewing all informed consent and liability release forms.

See the sidebar on page 112 for a sample informed consent form that you can modify for your needs. Additional risk management guidelines include the following:

- Making sure all exercise instructors, supervisors, and program directors are properly certified by a reputable organization
- Requiring all participants in high-risk activities to wear appropriate clothing and use appropriate equipment at all times
- Making sure all equipment and facilities such as spas, whirlpools, steam rooms, and tanning salons feature clear, easy-to-see instructions with precautionary warnings
- Explaining the possibility of injuries associated with aerobics, racquetball, weightlifting, and other activities to all participants before they participate
- Requiring participants to sign an informed consent form before participating
- Using only nationally recognized screening tests and procedures
- Developing and following a reliable injury reporting system
- Developing a hierarchy of supervision to ensure accountability for all phases of program and facility operations
- Designating who is responsible to whom and for what specific duties

Many smaller worksites do not have adequate personnel, facilities, and equipment to conduct appropriate preexercise screening. In such settings, a questionnaire can be helpful in assessing a person's cardiovascular health. Employees with any positive responses on the questionnaire should meet with their personal physician for further consultation and permission to exercise. You may use the questionnaire shown in the sidebar on page 112 or modify it as necessary.

Because health screening is both labor- and time-intensive, efficiency is particularly important for small businesses. Although most small businesses do not have in-house screening personnel, they can consider networking with local agencies by

- negotiating with the local health department to conduct a basic health screening for employees at little or no cost,
- arranging with a local health club for employees to receive a complimentary health screening in exchange for allowing the club to display its literature at the worksite,
- sponsoring an annual health fair and asking exhibitors to provide health screenings for employees, and
- asking faculty members (exercise physiologists, nurses, physical therapists, and health educators) at a local university to conduct employee health screenings in exchange for using their worksite as a possible research site.

# Sample Informed Consent Form

In consideration of my voluntary participation in (organization's name) health promotion program or any other activities sponsored by (organization) conducted on or off (organization) property, I hereby release and discharge (organization) from any and all claims for damages suffered by me as a result of my participation in these activities. I specifically release and discharge (organization) and its health promotion staff from all injuries or damages arising from or contributing to any physical impairment or defect I may have, whether latent or patent, and agree that (organization) is under no obligation to provide physical examination or other evidence of my fitness to participate in such activities, the same being my sole responsibility. Further, I understand that participation is not a condition of employment at (organization).

_____       _____
**Date**                          **Signature**

## Preactivity Screenings

| Date | Staff | Type | Results |
|------|-------|------|---------|
| _____ | _____ | _____ | _____ |
| _____ | _____ | _____ | _____ |
| _____ | _____ | _____ | _____ |

### Employee Health Status

____ Excellent

____ Good

____ Fair

____ Poor

____ Very Poor

### Activity Recommendation

____ Approved for participation

____ Approved, conditional

____ Rejected, further screening necessary

_____       _____
**Date**                          **Program Director**

# Sample Cardiovascular Screening Questionnaire

| Condition | Yes | No |
|-----------|-----|----|
| 1. Have you ever had a heart attack? | _____ | _____ |
| 2. Have you ever had a heart problem? | _____ | _____ |
| 3. Have you ever had "angina" (chest pain)? | _____ | _____ |
| 4. Were you born with a heart condition? | _____ | _____ |
| 5. Have you ever had high blood pressure? | _____ | _____ |
| 6. Have you ever had diabetes? | _____ | _____ |
| 7. Do you smoke? | _____ | _____ |
| 8. Have you ever had a thyroid condition? | _____ | _____ |
| 9. Have you ever had surgery in the past? | _____ | _____ |
| 10. Are you currently taking any medication? | _____ | _____ |
| 11. If you are female, are you pregnant? | _____ | _____ |

# GIVING THE PROGRAM A TRIAL RUN

As the planning process winds down and the program nears implementation, it's a good idea to conduct a trial run to identify potential problems and make necessary adjustments. It is especially good when planning a health fair or a new exercise program in order to assess traffic flow, space, equipment, facilities, and employee interest. You can conduct a trial run in four steps:

1. Recruit the number of employees you expect to participate at one time.
2. Explain the structure and purpose of the exercise facility and equipment and how to use the apparatus.
3. Have each person occupy a specific piece of equipment or station so that the entire facility is occupied.
4. Instruct all participants to exercise at their stations for a designated duration before proceeding to the next station.

As these steps are undertaken, check to see if the time allotted is enough for employees to successfully complete each routine. Is the transition smooth, or is it choppy? If you notice a delay, identify possible reasons for it and consider revising the facility layout or instructions for better efficiency.

## End-of-Program Rewards

As a program nears completion, WHP planners should be thinking ahead to the next program. Part of this involves motivating employees who have finished one program to pursue other programs that will benefit them. Here are some suggested rewards to give those employees who complete a program:

- Enter the employee in a company-wide sweepstakes or lottery. Draw one or more winners for prizes.
- Highlight employees with notable achievements in the company's newsletter.

- Designate a Wall of Fame to highlight employees who consistently set a good example for other employees.
- Offer employees with noteworthy improvements designated parking spaces at work for the month.
- Give away T-shirts that convey a specific theme or accomplishment at designated times (e.g., "I Kicked Butts" at the end of the smoking cessation program).
- Ask management to send a congratulatory letter to employees who complete a program.

## WHAT WOULD YOU DO?

Read the following four case studies. Then, choose one study to which to apply the strategies described in this chapter that are relevant to the following four components.

1. *Customer research*: How will you identify employee needs and interests?
2. *Marketing*: Create a marketing mix.
3. *Development and implementation*: Describe how you will develop and implement your program.
4. *Evaluation:* Describe what variables you will measure to determine program impact.

→ **Case Study 1:** A coal mine in New Mexico employs 85% Navajo American Indians. Total employee population is 375 people (90% men and 10% women). The mine is unionized and works three rotating 8-hour shifts. The mine has three different sites with separate entrances. The union participates in a nationwide health insurance plan negotiated specifically for coal miners, and it includes little preventive care. Management will only participate and pay for health promotion activities if employees drive the program.

→ **Case Study 2:** A refinery in the Gulf Coast employs 90% men and 10% women. The total employee population is 1,200, with an average age of 42. The nonunion plant requires 70% heavy labor work and two rotating 12-hour work shifts. A health promotion program has been in place for 2 years with an on-site fitness facility of 10,000 square feet. The top employee risk factors are poor eating habits, stress, back injuries, high blood cholesterol, and lack of exercise.

→ **Case Study 3:** In a large midwestern city, a cellular phone company has five worksites with 1,500 white-collar employees. The population is 50% male and 50% female, with an average age of 34. The majority of employees have a college education and the company is non-union. Access to health promotion and risk-reduction programs is limited to the choice of two managed care plans.

→ **Case Study 4:** Located on the East Coast are 55 offshore oil platforms, which house 15 to 40 employees at each bunkhouse. Each facility has a catered food arrangement, and 17 have functioning fitness facilities. The population is nonunion and 90% blue-collar males. The employees belong to a traditional indemnity (fee-for-service) health plan, and emergency room visits are the most common claim.

# Evaluating Health Promotion Efforts

After reading this chapter you will be able to

→ List several pitfalls that can compromise an evaluation.

→ Identify typical WHP program stakeholders by title and rationale for their interest in evaluation.

→ Distinguish between goals and objectives.

→ Give examples of process, impact, and outcome evaluation.

→ Explain the primary difference between a nonexperimental design and a quasi-experimental design.

**E**arly supporters of health promotion activities, particularly in the worksite, were personally committed to encouraging efforts in health promotion and disease prevention because they made sense. However, the time for blind acceptance of WHP's presumed effectiveness has passed. Some programs that have forgone evaluation of their programs in favor of investing those dollars in program activities are now in trouble or have ceased operations. Today, business leaders are asking for data-driven results to support the continuation of longstanding and, in some cases, expensive programs. Other organizations that are just establishing new programs are setting clear expectations for measurable outcomes.

With greater challenges to produce more results using limited resources, how can an organization know whether its WHP programs are on the right track? How do you show tangible proof that something is working? In large part, it depends on how decision makers approach program evaluation and on their ability to avoid common pitfalls that compromise the integrity of any evaluation. Some of the most common pitfalls include the following:

• *Having no goal or vision for doing an evaluation*: In other words, no clearly delineated concept of why an evaluation is needed, what components will comprise an evaluation, and who can benefit from the results exists.

• *Having unrealistic expectations*: For example, decision makers expect that a single evaluation will tell them exactly what they need to do to turn a substandard program into an award-winning program overnight.

• *Reaching no interdepartmental consensus on the scope and specificity of an evaluation*: For example, program managers differ on what to evaluate, how to conduct an evaluation, and how they will use the results.

• *Having inadequate financial resources*: Although 5% to 10% of a program budget is generally accepted as an appropriate level to devote to an evaluation, some evaluations require two or three times this level.

• *Inaccessibility to essential data or inability to obtain it*: For example, the human resources manager has not established a good rapport with the third-party administrator and, thus, is unable to obtain aggregate medical claims data in a timely manner.

• *Evaluating a program before its time*: For example, someone conducts a break-even analysis on a new fitness center after only several months of its opening.

• *Not having adequate resources in place*: For instance, no one makes a plan to secure appropriate data tools, equipment, and personnel in a timely manner.

• *Using an inappropriate evaluation design*: For example, no one makes an effort to include a matched group of nonparticipants to minimize the potential impact of external factors.

• *Not identifying all evaluation stakeholders*: For example, someone conducts an evaluation without considering who should receive the evaluation results; consequently, the scope and specificity of the actual evaluation is not applicable to key decision makers.

Most of these pitfalls relate to many factors for decision makers to consider in planning and conducting a program evaluation. Let's investigate how specific factors affect decisions in planning and conducting an evaluation. To cut this huge task down to size, it is important to approach an evaluation through decision points. A simple way to envision a decision point is to look at the questions listed in table 8.1.

# EVALUATION PLAN

Several decades ago, Edward Suchman, one of America's great social researchers, said this about program evaluation:

> All social institutions or subsystems—whether medical, educational, religious, economic, or political—are required to provide proof of their legitimacy and

**Table 8.1  Sample Decision Points in a Socratic-Based Evaluation Plan**

|  | Evaluation goals | Evaluation design | Evaluation objectives | Scope and specificity | Economics |
|---|---|---|---|---|---|
| What | What are the goals of this evaluation? | What target population will be evaluated? | What actions need to be taken to complete an evaluation? | What type of evaluation (process, impact, or outcome) is appropriate? | What types of benefit and cost variables are appropriate? |
| Why | Why are we evaluating this program? | Why are we using a particular design? |  | Why is a specific type of evaluation appropriate in this setting? |  |
| How | How were the goals established? | How long is the evaluation time frame? How will we collect data? |  | How precise a measurement should we use for the outcome variable? | How much will the evaluation cost? |
| When |  | When will measurements be performed? | When should each objective be completed? | When will we know if the evaluation is proceeding as originally planned? | When is a reasonable time frame to compare costs to benefits? |
| Where |  | Where will we conduct the evaluation? |  |  | Where can we obtain the funding for an evaluation? |
| Who |  | Who will conduct the evaluation? Who will analyze data? | Who is responsible for each objective? | Who should decide on the type of evaluation to use? |  |

effectiveness in order to justify society's continued support. Both the demand for and type of acceptable proof will depend largely on the nature of the relationship between the social institution and the public. In general, a balance will be struck between faith and fact, reflecting the degree of man's respect for authority and tradition within the particular system versus his skepticism and desire for tangible proof of work. (Suchman 1967, p. 1)

Perhaps Suchman's commentary can serve to remind us that any intervention needs substantiation.

To evaluate anything, you have to know what it is you are evaluating. Thus, the first thing to do when planning an evaluation is to identify all individuals who have a stake in knowing about the results of the program you are proposing to evaluate and to find out what they want to know. Once you understand what they are interested in, you can proceed with the task of developing appropriate evaluation goals. However, take this precaution: If you are either inexperienced or simply new to an organization, it may be very useful to do a quick informal survey of available resources before developing goals. By doing so, you can get some idea of what resources are likely to be available to guide your goal planning. Moreover, it will keep you from the extremes of

## Questions Addressed by Evaluation

- Can a WHP program provide measurable benefits to employees and an organization?
- To what extent do all participants benefit from a WHP program?
- How can we tell whether a program has more impact on direct benefits or indirect benefits?
- Can these programs really impact productivity measures such as absenteeism, presenteeism, on-the-job injury, and short-term disability?
- What types of programs are most cost-effective in a company with a demographic profile similar to our workforce?
- How long does it take for a program to break even?

being overly optimistic about what can be done or underestimating the possibilities.

Designing an evaluation cannot be done effectively unless you include input from the program stakeholders—those people who have something to gain or lose from the evaluation results. Thus, you must establish who the program stakeholders are and enlist their cooperation. Corporate financial officers, specific program managers (e.g., benefits, safety, risk management, loss prevention, and so on) health promotion staff members, program participants, and sponsors (if a funding source is involved) will probably all have questions they would like to have answered about the program. You will find that different stakeholders have different interests, and you must be sure to include evaluation goals that address all of their questions.

How can you be sure you have identified all the stakeholders? It will help to take these four factors into account:

1. The administrative structure of an organization's decision-making style
2. The rationale for doing an evaluation
3. The history and maturity of the program being evaluated
4. The political realities surrounding the evaluation

Each of these factors is important to consider. For example, suppose a WHP program director wanted an outside consulting firm to do a medical claims data analysis. The primary reason for doing the data analysis was to identify the percentage of employees' claim costs linked to smoking, physical inactivity, obesity, and other potentially modifiable risk factors. Based on the risk factor cost distributions from the analysis, appropriate programming and risk-reduction interventions could then be established by WHP staff. Although the director only requested that the analysis be prepared for her, the consultants suggested the report also be targeted to the human resources director and departmental representatives throughout the company.

*Here is how the four factors that can identify stakeholders affect this recommendation:*

1. The administrative structure of an organization's decision-making style: Through discussions with the WHP program director, the consultants discovered that she had requested that an evaluation should

address several employee health issues that had been identified initially by her boss, the human resources director. Clearly, the human resources director was a key decision maker in the program.

2. The rationale for doing an evaluation: Because the evaluation centered initially around risk factors, the consultants recognized that various health management personnel (e.g., occupational health, workers' compensation, safety, loss prevention, risk management, and so on) who were responsible for implementing specific risk-reduction programs may also wish to receive the evaluation results.

3. The history and maturity of the program being evaluated: The consultants learned that the WHP program was relatively new and that the program director was trying to expand it to reach a larger share of the workforce. This suggested to the consultants that it was important to apprise various departmental representatives of the program's current and future value, creating support throughout the company for the WHP program director's goal.

4. The political realities surrounding the evaluation: By recognizing that the human resources director and department heads had been very influential in establishing past and present program policies, it was clear to the consultants that without the support of these individuals, the expansion of the worksite health promotion program could not evolve.

When the consultants shared their concerns about customizing the report to the human resources director and the department heads, the program director quickly understood that expanding the audience for the report and addressing the concerns of major stakeholders would significantly enhance her ability to broaden the WHP program.

What kinds of questions will stakeholders have? Quite varied, in many cases. Program administrators may want to know what percentage of the program budget is spent on operational costs within the program. Health promotion staff members may want to know whether the newly enacted financial incentives are motivating high-risk employees to participate. Funding

sponsors may want to know whether their money produced some positive outcomes. The questions that stakeholders will want answered will be as numerous and varied as the people involved. Finding out all of these questions may take some ingenuity. Based on an organization's culture and decision-making style, it may be appropriate to call a meeting of key decision makers and brainstorm, distribute a written survey, or quiz them by phone or e-mail. Some companies hold an annual WHP staff planning retreat in which stakeholders are invited and asked to brainstorm with the staff on what programs and program evaluations they would like to see in the future.

## Health-Related Goals Versus Financial Goals

Goals of greatest interest to stakeholders are of two primary types: health-related and financial. If you neglect to include both categories of goals, you also neglect to plan for the evaluation types, designs, and instruments necessary to measure them. Evaluation helps determine whether health program goals and objectives are met and also answers questions about the program as it is being implemented. Thus, evaluation planning should be tied closely to the development of a program's goals and objectives. If these goals and objectives are designed with ease of evaluation in mind, then

• Assessments can be made easily during the course of the program, enabling staff members to improve the program as it progresses. For example, if ongoing evaluations are scheduled, WHP personnel might discover that the low enrollment in a stress management workshop reflects an inadequate location, inconvenient hours, ineffective marketing, or lack of publicity. These problems, once identified, could be addressed and eliminated.

• Clearly defined goals that are required of any evaluation can help program presenters and participants keep on track through ongoing mini-evaluations.

If the evaluation is not designed until the program has ended, neither of these benefits is possible. Moreover, carefully designed goals will enable you to focus on what the intervention can reasonably be expected to achieve, clarifying the impact of the intervention on its target.

Laudable as health-related goals may be, they cannot be pursued in isolation from financial goals. If money is not available to run WHP programs, the health-related goals can never be achieved. Thus, it is crucial that health-related goals be addressed within the limitations imposed by financial necessity. These limitations vary from organization to organization, depending on the financial resources of those organizations as well as on the values of those who control the purse strings.

Key decision makers holding the purse strings are usually interested in financial goals. They want to address questions that can be answered by using econometric-based evaluation tools such as break-even analysis, cost-effectiveness analysis, forecasting, and benefit-cost analysis.

## Intervention Goals

After you have established clearly delineated goals for doing an evaluation, you can proceed with developing goals for your program interventions. For example, what is the goal for your back health program? Because you are developing your evaluation goals in connection with specific programs, you must think not only about goals that are tied to evaluation but about the general goals of the programs as well. If the goals of those programs are properly developed, it makes your program intervention goals that much easier to develop as well. (Note that the following terms are used interchangeably: outcome variable, dependent variable, outcome, and goal.) Evaluation is greatly enhanced when the program it is evaluating contains goals that are developed according to five criteria:

1. *Compatibility with stakeholders' personal health and values:* Participants, program personnel, top management, or other stakeholders value the desirable outcome.
2. *Measurability:* Evaluators can physically or statistically measure changes that may occur in the outcome variable.
3. *Quantifiability:* Evaluators can track and attach a statistical value (e.g., #, $, %) to the outcome variable.
4. *Sufficient intervention time frame:* The intervention will be offered long enough to have a reasonable chance to influence the outcome variable.
5. *Realistically achievable:* Likelihood is high that the intervention is inherently strong enough to impact the outcome variable.

It is not uncommon to see organizational health promotion goals that lack one or more of the five criteria. An example of such an incomplete goal would be: "Within 1 year, hypertension-related medical costs will drop by at least 20%." Conversely, a goal that incorporates all five criteria would be: "Within 6 months [time frame], 60% [realistically achievable] of the male workforce [stakeholders] will have blood pressure readings of 130/85 or less [quantifiable] as measured during their physical exam [measurable]."

Let's take a couple of goals that are not very useful initially for either planning or evaluation and, by applying the five goal criteria, rewrite them until they are useful for evaluation. Suppose the following are your two goals:

1. Improve the cardiovascular health of female employees.
2. Improve employee productivity.

Now, one by one, here is how adding the elements defined in each of the criteria can transform these vaguely defined goals into valuable tools for planning both programs and evaluations.

### Compatibility With Stakeholders' Health or Values

When you create your goals, you must be certain that the stakeholders will support them. If you ran a survey of women in your workforce and learned that the primary health concern of 80% of them was to lessen their chances of breast cancer, you would have a hard time selling a cardiovascular health program, especially if it were ranked lower in preference. If you had limited funds and could afford only one major program for women, you would want to change the focus of your goal to reflect the women's primary interests.

You might rewrite your goals (including measurability and sufficient intervention time frame, as well as compatibility) the following way:

1. Reduce breast cancer risk levels among female employees.
2. Improve employee productivity.

You would have saved yourself some trouble had you surveyed the stakeholders in your women's health program before you decided on your goal. Assume that you had surveyed major stakeholders already about employee productivity; thus, that goal remains the same.

## Measurability and Quantifiability

Although both of your goals are now compatible with the interests of your stakeholders, neither is particularly useful yet because neither contains anything that can be measured. One way of stating this requirement for measurability would be to say that in order for a goal statement to be measurable, it must contain a dependent variable. Note that a dependent variable is an observable property that varies—that is, takes on different values—depending on the impact of the intervention (the independent variable) and to which numbers can be assigned. Examples of dependent variables are blood pressure level, sick-leave absenteeism, medical costs, and productivity.

The unacceptable goals listed previously can be improved by assigning to each of them a quantifiable dependent variable that could serve as a measurement of progress toward the general goal. For example:

1. "Reduce breast cancer risk levels among female employees as evidenced by at least a 20% reduction in the number of breast cancer–specific risk factors."
2. "Improve employee productivity through a 10% reduction in the number of unscheduled absences."

You can see that the second version of each goal includes a measurement factor. You can also see from the two preceding examples that it is not possible to write measurable program goals in the absence of baseline data. You cannot, after all, tell when an improvement in anything has occurred if you do not know the original level.

Thus, if no baseline exists for the area being measured, the first goal should be to establish one. For example, for the two sample goals, you would need to know the current breast cancer risk-factor status of the female workforce and something like the average absenteeism rates throughout the workforce for the last 3 years. In the case of certain program evaluation goals, a baseline value could be established in the first evaluation time frame.

## Sufficient Intervention Time Frame

To know how to plan and be able to evaluate, you must include some kind of time frame in your goals. For example:

1. Reduce breast cancer risk levels among female employees as evidenced by at least a 20% reduction in the number of breast cancer–specific risk factors within 6 months, and
2. Improve employee productivity through a 10% reduction in unscheduled absenteeism within 4 months.

Now you have a defined target at which you can aim. Without a definite deadline to aim for, your measurement of progress is not very meaningful. Only if you know how you're doing within a time frame can you know whether you need to change your intervention methods to be more effective or whether it would be reasonable to set your sights higher than your original goal.

## Realistic Achievability

It is important to establish a goal that is realistically achievable in order not to create false expectations for yourself or others. Although the goals developed so far are compatible with stakeholders' personal goals and feature both measurability and a sufficient intervention time frame, you must also be sure that they are realistic. How do you do this? By studying similar WHP programs and learning what their results have been as well as the factors that have affected their success rates, you can form a good idea of what is realistically achievable for your situation. In fact, some evaluation experts suggest that once you establish what seems like realistic goals, you should lower your sights a bit to take into account differences you may have overlooked.

Suppose you do your homework regarding the two goals we have been developing and discover that they are not realistic. Specifically, you learned that the original time lines were too ambitious compared to other case studies. Based on what you have learned, then, you revise your goals as follows:

1. Reduce breast cancer risk levels among female employees as evidenced by at least a 20% reduction in the number of breast cancer–specific risk factors within 1 year.
2. Improve employee productivity by reducing unscheduled absenteeism by at least 10% within 6 months.

If you have a general idea of what you would like to accomplish in your program, applying this four-step procedure to those general ideas will yield goals that are compatible with your stakeholders' interests and that are measurable, time-framed, and realistic.

## Establishing Measurable Objectives

Once program goals have been developed, it's time to establish measurable objectives to indicate what actions must be taken to achieve each goal. Objectives can be considered as steps or rungs in a ladder that enable program planners to achieve a particular goal. As you climb each rung (perform each objective), you are a step closer to reaching your goal. As an evaluator, you should be very interested in objectives because properly written objectives will facilitate and enhance the quality of the evaluation process and results. To be most valuable for program planners and evaluators, objectives should be

- tangible or visible,
- measurable,
- relevant to the goal, and
- implemented within a designated time frame.

When constructing objectives, you should do the following:

- *Establish short-term objectives to use in monitoring progress in the initial phase of the intervention.* For example: "At the end of one month, at least 75% of all original participants will be actively involved in personalized risk-reduction programs."

- *Establish midterm objectives to use in monitoring progress midway in an intervention.* For example: "At the end of three months, at least 65% of all original participants will be actively involved in personalized risk-reduction programs."

- *Establish long-term objectives to determine if midway progress has been sustained.* For example: "At the end of 6 months, at least 50% of all original participants achieving their initial risk-reduction goals will have maintained or exceeded that level of success."

- *Avoid the temptation to establish a long list of objectives, especially if the intervention to be evaluated is short-term, evaluations have not been conducted in the past, or an evaluation will be used as a prelude to a more formalized and thorough evaluation to be conducted later.* Too many objectives can add unnecessary procedures that increase the cost of conducting an evaluation.

- *Specify time frames when appropriate.* For example: "All participants will be screened on a quarterly basis at a minimum, and more frequently if they are classified as high risk."

Properly written objectives are invaluable in planning the evaluation process. Suppose, for example, that the primary goal of a prenatal health program is to reduce the number of pregnancy complications by at least 20% within 12 months as compared to the previous year. Following are specific objectives relevant to this goal, followed by appropriate evaluation planning decisions you might make based on that objective.

- **Objective 1.** Identify the target population (all female employees and female dependents). Evaluation planning decision: During weeks 1 through 4, contact the employer's insurer or claims administrator to obtain medical claims data for identifying the number of pregnancy complications.

- **Objective 2.** Conduct an analysis of pregnancy claims data from the past 2 years to identify specific types of pregnancy-related complications; review specific complications by their respective ICD (International Classification of Disease) or DRG (Diagnostic-Related Group). Evaluation planning decision: During weeks 5 and 6, develop a framework for recording the number of each type of complication that occurred in the past 2 years.

- **Objective 3.** Develop an expanded prenatal screening and prenatal health education program with financial incentives. Evaluation planning decision: During weeks 7 and 8, develop a framework to track participation in the screening and during the program.

- **Objective 4.** Inform all women of the new program and incentives using bulletin boards, paycheck stuffers, e-mail, and newsletters. Evaluation planning decision: During weeks 9 and 10, prepare an appropriate strategy to distribute each informational tool.

- **Objective 5.** Provide orientation sessions, including a comprehensive health screening, to identify women at risk for pregnancy complications. Construct a baseline data format. Evaluation planning decision: During weeks 11 and 12, establish an evaluation design, e.g., two-group quasi-experimental design in which participants serve as the experimental group and nonparticipants serve as the comparison group.

• **Objective 6.** Initiate on-site programs and additional referrals to personal physicians for selected women, if necessary. Evaluation planning decision: During weeks 13 through 18, record the names and number of on-site participants and off-site referrals.

• **Objective 7.** Monitor health status of at-risk women at appropriate (risk-based) intervals; provide customized interventions for each woman. Evaluation planning decision: During weeks 24 through 30, compare baseline health status levels against 6-month and 1-year levels. Analyze interval-to-interval changes to determine the intervention impact.

Another way to approach developing program objectives is to think about the items within the goal that you want to evaluate, then restate them as tasks rather than objectives. For example, suppose your goal is to reduce the direct cost of low-back injuries among warehouse and shipping department employees by 20% within 18 months. First, develop the following items to be measured:

• Total medical claims associated with low-back injuries

• Total participation as a percentage of the eligible population

• Total number of departmental supervisors who qualify for bonuses, based on program participation or enhanced productivity by their employees

• Total number of injury-free work hours by program participants

Based on this list of items, your program objective tasks would be as follows:

1. Conduct an analysis of medical claims associated with low-back injuries among warehouse and shipping department employees to identify the most common causes of injury.

2. Develop a low-back injury prevention program based on results of the claims analysis.

3. Develop an incentive program for participation; include incentives for both workers and supervisors.

4. Measure program participation.

5. Measure changes in workforce productivity.

6. Compare the total number of injury-free work hours among program participants and nonparticipants.

# EVALUATING TO PRODUCE INFORMATION

Some evaluators make the mistake of planning an evaluation after a WHP program is under way rather than in the planning phase. In these cases, evaluation procedures are often rushed and off base, resulting in unreliable results. Good planning gives evaluators enough time to properly lay out important elements of an evaluation, such as the following:

• What variables to measure

• What subjects to target

• Who conducts the evaluation

• How much financial support is needed

• When the evaluation should be conducted

• What evaluation equipment and instruments are needed

• What type of evaluation design is most appropriate

• How to use the results

• Who should have access to the results

As an evaluator, you should incorporate six basic guidelines in addressing each of these elements:

1. Have some idea of what type of outcome results you are looking for. Decide what factors and outcomes are most important to track.

2. Be in a position to act on the results. Secure management support and form alliances with specific departments in order to obtain essential data (safety, medical, benefits, and human resources, in particular).

3. Follow scientifically sound statistical procedures that are appropriate for the scope and specificity of your evaluation. For example, will a t-test be sufficient to compare pre- and post-program results? What type of regression analysis is necessary to properly identify the relationships between several variables at the same time? Were previous cost savings adjusted to reflect today's market value?

4. Be able to differentiate normal from abnormal results. A slight drop in absenteeism

among program participants may be normal, but a 100% quit rate among smokers would be unrealistic.

5. Closely monitor each variable being measured. Are participants as satisfied with their personal coach now as they were on the first day? How many participants are losing body weight at a healthy rate? What types of health care claims have changed the most by ranking in the past year?

6. Convert data into valuable information, when possible. Identify and record any evolving trends by age, gender, risk-factor level, and so on. What implications can you extract from the results for future WHP programs, marketing strategies, health plan benefits, financial incentives, and so on?

## EVALUATION CATEGORIES

As you establish your evaluation framework, it is important to consider how the results of your evaluation will be used. An initial step in developing your framework should involve a technique to categorize your overall evaluation. It is common to find proponents of the process, impact, and outcome approach while others advocate the formative and summative approach. While both of these approaches can be applied in WHP evaluations, the author prefers the former approach primarily because it provides a three-tiered evaluation time frame designed to provide evaluators with more opportunities to scrutinize an intervention from start to finish.

**Process** evaluation focuses on what is happening during a program and specific aspects of the intervention that need attention. It can focus on either qualitative or quantitative questions.

Qualitative issues include aspects of program delivery such as program registration, educational content, and instructor effectiveness. For example, by looking at the age, gender, and job classification of employees who have participated in various program offerings, the evaluator can see whether one delivery mode, teaching method, instructor, or incentive appears to have drawn certain segments of the workforce more effectively than another. Reactions from participants about programming schedules, health screening procedures, fitness center hours, or workshop speakers could show program administrators what changes might be necessary to improve participation rates. The tools of qualitative analysis include short ques-

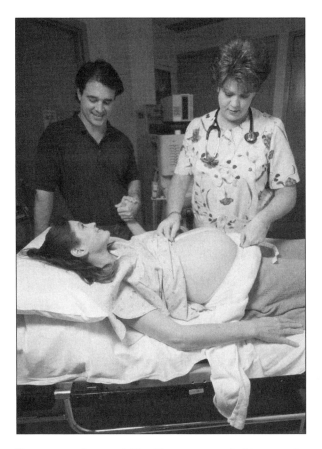

The success of a prenatal health program can first be gauged by process evaluation (e.g., instructor or class time popularity), then impact evaluation (e.g., reduction in pregnancy complications), and finally the outcome evaluation (e.g., a reduction in pregnancy complication costs).

tionnaires, personal solicitation, focus groups, suggestion boxes, e-mail communications, and other on-site media.

Using process evaluation can also address financial issues. Predicting when the break-even point will be, how much the cost savings will be, and when cost savings are realized can tell program administrators whether they should scale back or expand their original plans.

As an intermediate strategy, **impact** evaluation assesses the overall effectiveness of a program in producing desirable levels of knowledge, attitudes, behaviors, health status, and skills in a target population. For example: How many people stopped smoking? How many people can successfully perform CPR? How many people practice medical self-care? Essentially, changes in worksite behaviors, attitudes, and cultural norms are measured by impact evaluation using one or more survey techniques to compare pre- and postprogram status.

Common impact evaluation tools include

- questionnaires,
- health risk appraisals,
- health care claims data reports,
- occupational injury reports,
- absenteeism logs,
- culture audits (i.e., observing the worksite environment), and
- productivity or quality reports.

Considered the back-end or bottom-line strategy along the evaluation continuum, **outcome** evaluation determines and quantifies cost savings that may occur when an intervention affects absenteeism, productivity, health care utilization, and the like. Outcome evaluation focuses on the question, Did the intervention cause the changes that occurred and, if so, was the cost justifiable? For example, did the intervention

- reduce the blood pressure and medication usage resulting in lower medication costs?
- decrease the prevalence of stress-related counseling sessions and associated costs?
- improve communication between the benefits and medical departments and, thereby, increase interdepartmental efficiency and lower overall administration costs?
- decrease the incidence of low-back pain among program participants and result in a reduction of doctor visits, workers' compensation claims, and medical care costs?

Commonly used instruments of outcome evaluation include health claim cost reports, monthly expense reports, quarterly productivity reports, cost-effectiveness analysis, and benefit-cost analysis.

While process, impact, and outcome evaluation options are being considered in planning an evaluation, it is a good time to consider the rigor of an evaluation expected by the stakeholders. In today's budget-minded economy, many WHP program directors find themselves having to constantly justify their programs. Consequently, the scope of an evaluation must be designed to show that any changes are primarily caused by a WHP intervention while minimizing the potential effect that outside factors such as the media, corporate policies, and societal changes may have on the actual outcome. While it is impossible to completely eliminate the influence of media and societal forces on human health, WHP evalua-

tors should use appropriate evaluation designs to establish a reasonable level of rigor and objectivity in their quest to do so. Let's take a look at several options for WHP personnel to consider when selecting an evaluation design.

# EVALUATION DESIGN

An evaluation design includes the following essential components (see table 8.2):

- **Experimental group (E):** The group of employees that participate in the program.
- **Control or comparison group (C):** A control group that consists of employees who are similarly matched to the experimental group of employees participating in the intervention; in contrast, a comparison group consists of persons who are not matched (nonequivalent) to the experimental group.
- **Observation (O):** When a measurement is performed.
- **Independent variable (X):** The program intervention designed to produce a positive outcome.

**Table 8.2 Major Parts of a Sample Evaluation Design**

|  | E | C |
| --- | --- | --- |
| First measurement (observation) | $O_1$ | $O_1$ |
| Program | X |  |
| Second measurement | $O_2$ | $O_2$ |

Evaluation designs vary significantly in their scope and specificity, so you will need to tailor your design to the specific needs and interests of your worksite. Several examples of program evaluation design follow.

## Nonexperimental Design

Nonexperimental designs (table 8.3) represent basic and relatively weak designs that, in real worksite settings, may be the only viable option when evaluators cannot assign participants to an experimental or control group, or there is no comparison group. The most basic nonexperimental design is the one-group pretest and posttest design. This design consists of a single measurement before a program is implemented

### Table 8.3 Two Common Nonexperimental Designs

| Pretest-posttest | Time series |
|---|---|
| E | E |
| $O_1$ | $O_1$ |
|  | $O_2$ |
|  | $O_3$ |
| X | X |
|  | $O_4$ |
|  | $O_5$ |
| $O_2$ | $O_6$ |

and a second evaluation at the end of the program. This design is easy to conduct in worksite settings but has two major drawbacks:

1. Because no measurement is taken during the program, evaluators have to wait until the end of the program to determine whether the program made an impact.
2. Because no comparison or control group exists, various factors such as weather

conditions, a change in company policy, a change in work responsibilities, a change in personal health status, and so on could actually influence the outcome more than the intervention. Without a control or comparison group (which may also be likely to exercise more in good weather), it is difficult to measure the true impact of a fitness or weight management intervention because it was supplemented with personal exercise.

*Essentially, in these types of situations, we have to ask whether the results were influenced by*

- extraneous events, such as a television program or public campaign that occurred between $O_1$ and $O_2$ that may have influenced the subjects' behavior,
- the growth and development of subjects that occur with the mere passage of time between $O_1$ and $O_2$,
- the effect of $O_1$ on $O_2$ (that is, the pretest could have sensitized the subjects to what to expect in the posttest),
- changes in the measurement tools or procedures between $O_1$ and $O_2$, or

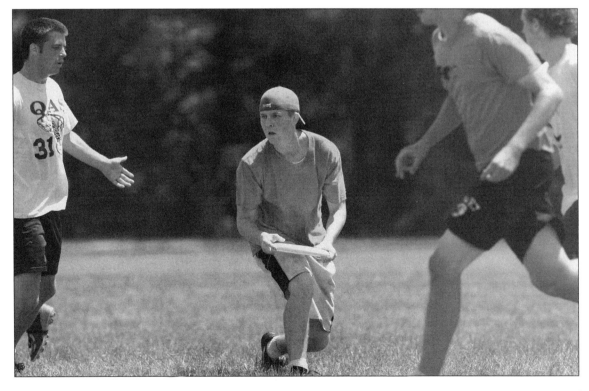

Pleasant weather might motivate more fitness program participants to exercise on their own, impacting the results of the intervention.

- interaction between the pretest and the program intervention. For example, the pretest itself may influence a person's behavior by making the participant aware of things they should or should not do.

Because outside forces can interfere with an intervention, evaluators should try to add a comparison group in their evaluation efforts. This would expand the scope of the nonexperimental design to that of a quasi-experimental design.

Presumably, the comparison group and the experimental group would have exercised the same amount outside of work, on average, and so would have experienced equal or similar benefits from any additional exercise they did on their own. Thus, the difference between the two groups in the amount of weight lost could be directly attributed to the worksite weight management program.

Despite their inherent drawbacks, nonexperimental designs remain popular at many worksites, especially in programs with very limited resources or small numbers of participants. In some cases, logistical constraints prevail, and a shorter-than-usual intervention makes it impractical to recruit a comparison group. Regardless, the point is that an evaluation generally has more credibility when a comparison group can be included.

## Quasi-Experimental Design

A type of evaluation design commonly used in WHP settings is the quasi-experimental design (see table 8.4). The prefix *quasi* means almost or nearly. Thus, a quasi-experimental design is similar to, but not as strong as, a true experimental design because of limitations in the random selection and random assignment of subjects to specific interventions. Although these designs can be used to show evidence of a program's effectiveness, they cannot control for all factors that influence the actual outcome of a WHP intervention. Moreover, no random assignment of subjects to either the experimental group (participants) or comparison group (nonparticipants) exists.

The pretest-posttest design is often used when a control group cannot be formed by random assignment. In such cases, a comparison group (a nonequivalent control group) is identified, and both groups are measured before and after the program. For example, you could use a pre- and postprogram fitness test to evaluate a fitness

program. Employees volunteering to participate in the program would comprise the experimental group while the remaining employees could serve as the comparison group. Because a strong likelihood exists that volunteers are already more physically active and more fit than nonvolunteers, we can assume an initial difference between the groups on their pretest fitness tests. Thus, in order to achieve more equality between the two groups, it is necessary to identify nonparticipants with similar baseline levels of fitness as the participants. You can identify them through matching (see the following section for an example of matching).

One of the stronger quasi-experimental evaluation frameworks is the multiple time series (MTS) design. It is structured as the true experimental time series design, but it uses a nonequivalent comparison group. This design can be extended in the same way a staggered evaluation design is, adding more posttests for the two groups, adding experimental groups to examine variations in the program, or both.

**Table 8.4 Two Common Quasi-Experimental Designs**

| Pretest-posttest | | Time series | |
|---|---|---|---|
| E | C | E | C |
| $O_1$ | $O_1$ | $O_1$ | $O_1$ |
| | | $O_2$ | $O_2$ |
| | | $O_3$ | $O_3$ |
| X | | X | |
| | | $O_4$ | $O_4$ |
| | | $O_5$ | $O_5$ |
| $O_2$ | $O_2$ | $O_6$ | $O_6$ |

This design is especially suited for evaluators who have access to past (retrospective) and future (prospective) data or who can conduct measurements on a regular basis. For example, suppose a company has established a voluntary back-stretching program to reduce the prevalence and cost of back injuries. Various types of MTS designs can be used to evaluate the program, assuming evaluators can measure the number of low-back injuries that occurred before, during, and after the program. Measurements are taken before the program to determine whether one group is noticeably different from the other group. By comparing any change in the number of back injuries among participants ($O_1$ to $O_2$) to any change in the number of back injuries among nonparticipants ($O_1$ to $O_2$), evaluators can compare injury rates between the two groups before the program. In addition, they can compare injury data for both groups a second time ($O_2$ to $O_3$) to give evaluators greater insight about any possible preprogram differences between the groups. If one group shows significantly fewer back injuries than the other group before the program, evaluators can select a second group of nonparticipants for comparison. This comparison group ideally has a similar number of back injuries to the participant group. If not, evaluators can choose a third group of nonparticipants and so on, until a comparison group with back-injury risks similar to the experimental group is identified.

Random assignment is not required in MTS designs, so it is possible for participants to be inherently different from nonparticipants. For example, suppose a risk manager suspects that a high percentage of employees are using a local hospital's emergency department for minor (nonemergency) conditions. A review of health care claims shows 75% of suspected emergency department abuses were incurred by employees under 40 years of age. While in the process of planning a new medical self-care program to attack this problem, the company distributed surveys on three preprogram occasions ($O_1$, $O_2$, and $O_3$) to assess employee interest in a self-care program. Suppose employees who expressed the highest interest in the program on the first occasion ($O_1$) also reported the most visits to the emergency department over the past year. Yet, on the second ($O_2$) and third ($O_3$) occasions, responding employees reportedly had the lowest rate of emergency department visits. By assessing employee interest on three separate occasions before implementing a self-care program, worksite health personnel were able to see that employees interested in the self-care program actually represented a broad cross section of employees. They could then use this information to determine whether a self-care program should be offered to the entire workforce or directed primarily toward employees under 40.

To minimize the possibility of having significant preprogram differences, evaluators should try to match participants and nonparticipants as closely as possible, especially on attributes linked with the outcome variable being measured. For example, various worksite studies suggest that an employee's risk of experiencing a back injury is influenced by these factors:

Age

Type of job

Body weight

Exercise habits

History of back injury

Job rotation opportunities

Prework stretching

Lifting habits

Abdominal strength

Hamstring and low-back flexibility

Work satisfaction

Stress level

An effective matching technique is to select (randomly, if possible) nonparticipating employees to form a comparison group that resemble participants. For example, if a new back-injury prevention program is being implemented, consider matching the groups on as many criteria related to back-injury risk. Because it is highly unlikely that you can choose nonparticipants that will closely match participants on all relevant criteria, you can establish a legitimate comparison group if it has some overall resemblance to participants. In essence, it is usually necessary to establish an acceptable range for specific criteria (table 8.5).

Once you develop acceptable ranges for each criterion, you must decide on a minimum number of acceptable criteria that nonparticipants have to meet in order to be included in the comparison group.

Another way to equate various groups is to randomly assign participants to different versions of a program. Random assignment is feasible when a new program has been added to an existing program or when a new program has two or more versions offered simultaneously. Say, for example, you have 50 employees sign up for a smoking cessation program. You can randomly divide the volunteers into two subgroups of 25 each, then show one group a self-help video and request the other group to attend on-site seminars (see table 8.6). Because the groups are selected

**Table 8.5  Acceptable Ranges of Criteria Related to Back-Injury Risk**

| Criteria | Participants | Nonparticipants |
|---|---|---|
| Work location | Warehouse | Warehouse |
| Average age | 37 yr | 35-40 yr |
| Average body weight | 185 lb (84 Kg) | 175-195 lb (80-89 kg) |
| Past back injuries | 1.5 per person | 1 to 2 |
| Exercise habits | 1.0 mi/day (1.6 km/day) | 0.5-1.5 mi/day (.08-2.4 km/day) |
| Rotate jobs | Do not | Do not |
| Prework stretch | Do not | Do not |
| Lifting habits | 15 lifts/day | 10-20 lifts/day |
| Abdominal strength | >15 sit-ups/min | >12 sit-ups/min |
| Work satisfaction | 80% of time | >70% of time |
| High stress level | 50% of time | >40% of time |

from one pool of volunteers, less chance exists that one group is significantly different from the other group. This design also allows evaluators to compare one particular intervention with another intervention to determine which is most cost-effective.

**Table 8.6  Multiple-Time Series Design With Two Randomly Assigned Groups**

| R | R |
|---|---|
| $E_1$ (Self-help video) | $E_2$ (On-site seminars) |
| $O_1$ | $O_1$ |
| $O_2$ | $O_2$ |
| $O_3$ | $O_3$ |
| X | X |
| $O_4$ | $O_4$ |
| $O_5$ | $O_5$ |
| $O_6$ | $O_6$ |

R = random assignment.

## Experimental Design

The most powerful type of evaluation design is the experimental design, in which participants are (a) randomly selected and (b) randomly assigned to experimental and control groups. An experimental design offers the greatest control over outside factors that may interfere with the intervention. Potential disadvantages of the experimental design are that they require a relatively large number of subjects in which to assign and that the intervention may have to be delayed for those in the control group. Moreover, they are typically time- and labor-intensive designs and may require informed consent from participants. Perhaps the main challenge for evaluators is that such designs have to be applied under highly controlled conditions in which the behavioral circumstances may be unnatural or unusual. For example, people who participate in a program that encourages a change in behavior (e.g., exercising more, eating less fat, or reducing television viewing) may experience greater stress and thus behave differently than they normally do. Therefore, evaluation outcomes may not be easily applicable to other organizational settings. Simply put, the rigorous procedures of an experimental design may increase the validity of the results, but they may have limited feasibility and generalizability. Table 8.7 illustrates various experimental designs.

Because evaluation designs vary significantly in their rigor and utility, you need to tailor your design to the specific needs and interests of your worksite. As you do so, take time to check that you are addressing all of the Socratic elements listed previously in table 8.1. As you prepare your evaluation and select an appropriate design, consider the scope and specificity of your evaluation needs and plan accordingly.

**Table 8.7  Experimental Designs**

| Pretest-Posttest | | Posttest only | | Time series | | Staggered treatment | | | |
|---|---|---|---|---|---|---|---|---|---|
| R | R | R | R | R | R | R | R | R | R |
| E | C | C | E | E | C | E1 | E2 | E3 | E4 |
| $O_1$ | $O_1$ | | | $O_1$ | $O_1$ | X | $O_1$ | $O_1$ | X |
| | | | | $O_2$ | $O_2$ | $O_1$ | X | X | $O_1$ |
| | | | | $O_3$ | $O_3$ | $O_2$ | $O_2$ | $O_2$ | |
| X | | | X | X | X | $O_3$ | $O_3$ | $O_3$ | |
| | | | | | $O_4$ | $O_4$ | $O_4$ | $O_4$ | |
| | | | | | $O_5$ | $O_5$ | | | |
| $O_2$ | $O_2$ | $O_1$ | $O_1$ | $O_4$ | $O_6$ | | | | |

# SCOPE AND SPECIFICITY

The structure of your evaluation plan is influenced largely by the scope and specificity of your evaluation needs. Scope refers to the range of variables and the time frame of the evaluation. For example, an evaluation consisting of several variables that are measured over a 1-year time frame has a broader scope than an evaluation involving one or two variables spanning 6 months. In contrast, specificity refers to the level or degree of precision evaluators use in measuring selected variables within an evaluation.

The number of variables you choose to look at and the time frame in which you do so will define the scope of your evaluation. For example, the scope of a back-injury prevention program evaluation will probably be smaller than a medical self-care program evaluation. Why? Because the back-program evaluation is more likely to focus on a single variable (number of back injuries) that can be influenced in a relatively short time, whereas the medical self-care program is likely to include several variables (e.g., number of self-care procedures, number of physician visits, medical care costs) that usually take longer to monitor in addition to taking longer to be influenced by the intervention.

In addition to establishing the scope of your evaluation, it is important to consider the specificity, or level of precision, that is appropriate for defining outcome variables. For example, an outcome variable such as absenteeism has virtually no level of specificity because it does not delineate specific types of (or reasons for) absenteeism. In contrast, an outcome variable stated as absenteeism related to low-back injuries has some level of specificity because it specifies why absences occurred. Programs that include outcome variables with a high level of specificity are generally preferred because they provide evaluators with greater opportunities to closely study the real impact of an intervention on a specific outcome variable (table 8.8).

Defining highly specific variables is only possible if problems and needs are carefully analyzed

**Table 8.8  Outcome Variables With Low and High Levels of Specificity**

| Variable | Less specificity | More specificity |
|---|---|---|
| Absenteeism | (All causes) | Caused by sick leave |
| Health care claims | Total number | Number by type of claim |
| Participation | Per month | Per week |
| High-risk employees | Total number | Number by age and gender |
| Injuries | Total cost | Average cost by type |

## Simplify!

A midsize utility company had been experiencing double-digit health care cost inflation over the past few years. Health managers reviewed several years of claims data and noticed that emergency department (ED) utilization was the fastest-growing claim during this time frame and that 35- to 45-year-old women had the highest ED usage, followed closely by 25- to 35-year-old men. The identified group of women worked primarily in the customer service department while the targeted group of males worked in the line repair division. Small group sessions with both groups were conducted to identify what factors were causing higher ED usage among these particular groups. Both groups indicated similar reasons for their ED usage: Many customer complaints reported in the late afternoon required customer service representatives to stay on the job beyond their scheduled 5 p.m. quitting time and thus prevented them from seeking care from their health care providers whose offices closed at 6 p.m.; and many line repairmen used the ED because they often worked overtime because of late-afternoon power failures. A final review of the individual ED claims by the occupational

health nurse indicated that virtually all of the health problems prompting ED visits were not emergencies, but minor ailments such as colds, sore muscles, and skin rashes. Realizing they could do little to influence the timing of customer complaints and power shortages, health managers decided to try reducing ED visits by teaching and motivating employees to treat minor ailments through a medical self-care (MSC) program. The health management staff established a program goal of reducing the number of ED visits associated with minor ailments by 25% within 1 year, based on their review of MSC program results reported in the professional literature. The MSC program included weekly small-group seminars during an expanded lunch period. By taking into consideration each target group's work schedule and health problems, staff members were able to establish an appropriate scope (selecting the fastest-growing claims and allowing ample time for the MSC program to have an effect before evaluating it) and specificity (zeroing in on only nonemergency ailments) for the program-dependent variables, ensuring among other things that the program could reasonably be evaluated.

early in the evaluation process. The example above shows how one company wrote a dependent variable with a high degree of specificity based on a careful examination of various factors affecting their rising health care costs. At the time when considering scope and specificity issues, evaluators should also take stock of the need for an economic-based evaluation.

# ECONOMIC-BASED EVALUATIONS

Two of the most common economic-based evaluations used in various worksites are cost-effectiveness analysis (CEA) and benefit-cost analysis (BCA)

## Cost-Effectiveness Analysis

What if program planners want to compare one program with another program to decide which one produces the greatest benefit for the least expense? Properly implemented, cost-effectiveness analysis (CEA) can answer that question. Rather than assigning monetary values

to a single outcome of a program, as is done in some analyses, CEA compares only the costs of similar programs for achieving a specific outcome. For example, if you wanted to know which smoking cessation programs were the most cost-effective, you could implement the CEA framework shown in table 8.9. The data in table 8.9 suggest the "cold turkey" program was less costly to provide at this worksite and three times more economical (or, one third as costly) as the gradual withdrawal approach. Conducting a CEA in a worksite setting involves several key steps:

1. Plan your evaluation as you plan your interventions.

   • Determine your program goals and objectives. Ask yourself what your interventions are supposed to do for employees and the organization. For example, the goal of your back program may be to prevent low-back injuries. Objectives listed in table 8.10 represent several activities that must be accomplished to achieve that goal. For example, the first and second objectives include screening as many employees as possible in the yearlong program. The third objective is to recruit and involve as many at-risk employees as possible in the yearlong program. The fourth and final objective is to obtain feedback from participants as to whether or not they had incurred a low-back injury during the intervention. The final objective listed in a CEA framework should reflect the main goal (desired outcome) of the intervention.

- Set up thorough record-keeping procedures. Consider major cost items such as personnel, facilities, and equipment; and minor cost items such as photocopying, printing, and record keeping.
- Determine the time frame in which you will compare the interventions.

2. *Calculate total costs for each intervention.* During the trial period, keep careful records following the procedures that you established in step one. At the end of the trial period, add up all expenses to arrive at the total cost for each intervention during that period.

3. *Determine the cost per outcome for each program intervention by dividing the cost of the program intervention by the number of quantitative units (impacts) listed within each objective.*

4. *Compare the final cost per outcome values for each program intervention and determine which is most cost-effective (see table 8.10).* Although the seminar and belt combination program initially costs five times as much as the daily stretch intervention, the stretch routine produced a higher return on investment. The daily stretch protected employees against a back injury at nearly one-seventh ($20/$135) the cost of the seminar and belt combination.

**Table 8.9  A Cost-Effectiveness Analysis Framework Used in Comparing Two Different Smoking Cessation Interventions**

| Type of program | Cost of program | PARTICIPANTS | | SUCCESSFUL QUITTERS | |
| --- | --- | --- | --- | --- | --- |
| | | Number of | Cost per | Number of | Cost per* |
| "Cold turkey" with self-help booklet | $2,000 | 100 | $20 | 50 | $40 |
| Gradual withdrawal with on-site counselor | $3,000 | 100 | $30 | 25 | $120 |

*Cost of program divided by number of successful quitters.

**Table 8.10  A Cost-Effectiveness Analysis of Two Worksite Programs**

| Program | Cost/year | Procedure/outcome | Cost/outcome |
| --- | --- | --- | --- |
| Monthly back seminar with lumbar belt | $5,000 | 100 screenings | $50 per screen |
| | | 50 diagnosed as high risk because of poor back flexibility or abdominal weakness | $100 per positive find |
| | | 40 participated | $125 per participant |
| | | 37 reported no low-back injury in first year of program | $135 per positive outcome |
| Daily prework stretching | $1,000 | 100 screenings | $10 per screen |
| | | 80 diagnosed as high risk because of poor back flexibility or abdominal weakness | $12.50 per positive find |
| | | 75 participated in daily stretching | $13.33 per participant |
| | | 50 reported no low-back injury within 1 year of program | $20 per positive find |

Although a CEA may show one program having a greater return on investment than another program, the decision to eliminate a particular program should not be based solely on this comparison alone. After all, a program with a moderate return on investment may produce benefits that are not easily quantified (e.g., enhanced employee morale and better management–labor relations).

## Benefit-Cost Analysis

The primary purpose of a benefit-cost analysis (BCA) is to determine whether a program is worth its cost. Because the BCA method compares program benefits to program costs, it might be most effective to measure both benefits and costs in monetary terms. However, some researchers caution that quantification should not be the sole basis for performing a benefit-cost analysis, contending that important factors should not be neglected just because they cannot be tangibly measured. For example, how would we quantify the suffering of people with severe back pain or chronic depression? Benefit-cost analysis doesn't purport to introduce rigor and quantification when the data are imprecise or where quantification is not feasible. However, when benefit and cost can be quantified, a BCA is a simple and efficient way to evaluate a program's success or value.

Because benefit-cost analysis provides meaningful data only to the extent that current or future benefits and costs can be accurately measured or projected, the first step in executing a BCA is to identify and measure benefits and costs as precisely as possible.

The cost side of a benefit-cost analysis involves calculating the costs of all resources such as personnel, equipment, and facilities used in planning and implementing an intervention. Table 8.11 shows typical direct and indirect costs.

The benefit side of the equation involves calculating the monetary value of any positive outcomes that can be quantified. As with costs, it is necessary to take both direct and indirect benefits into account. Indirect benefits are often referred to as opportunity benefits because they represent a financial resource that unexpectedly becomes available to invest in other interventions. Benefits, whether direct or indirect, include less health care utilization, lower medical costs, fewer accidents, lower absenteeism, and higher productivity. The effects of direct benefits are usually measurable using standard accounting

**Table 8.11 Typical Items on the Cost Side of a Benefit-Cost Analysis**

| Direct | Indirect |
| --- | --- |
| Medical care | Absenteeism (injured or sick employees) |
| Medical supplies | Additional tasks for coworkers |
| Medications | Training of replacement workers |
| Rehabilitation | Supervision of replacement workers |
| Employee assistance | Lower productivity of replacement workers |
| Workers' compensation | Data processing and administration |
| Case management | Overtime pay |
| ADA accommodations | Unexpected costs |

reports and conventional financial analysis. Before calculating any direct benefit, evaluators must identify an outcome (dependent) variable that can be treated as a direct benefit. In doing so, recall that a variable must be both measurable and relevant to the intervention.

After measuring all costs and identifying and measuring the value of all benefits, you can compare the two categories. To do this comparison, use either the net benefit method or the benefit-cost ratio method.

In the net benefit method, the evaluator determines the net benefit of a particular intervention and compares it with its cost. If the difference is positive, the analysis reveals that the intervention is financially worth the effort. The net benefit of any intervention may be calculated as follows:

$$\text{Net benefit} = [L\$ + GP + PI] - C$$

where

• L\$ (sometimes called the direct benefit) stands for the reduction in medical care expenses because of reduced risk, disease, or disability. For example, if the incidence of low-back injury declines, then some of the spending on health care services will no longer be necessary and, thus, available to employees, the employer, society, and other stakeholders.

• GP stands for the increase in general productivity, leading to greater output and income.

For example, if we reduce the incidence of low-back injury, we also increase the performance capabilities of the persons involved so they may continue to produce at desirable levels.

• PI stands for the gain in working income because of reduced injury and illness and their effects on absenteeism. GP and PI are the indirect benefits.

• C stands for the cost of the intervention.

For example, suppose an organization is experiencing a significant increase in low-back injury costs and responds by establishing a back-injury prevention program. After 6 months of the program, evaluators conduct a benefit-cost analysis. To use the formula provided, they need to find out the value of the reduction in medical care expenses related to low-back injuries, the increase in general productivity, and the drop in the cost of absenteeism that was initially traced to low-back injury. Here is what they find:

• Medical care expenses for back injuries have dropped from $125,000 to $35,000, so L$ = $90,000.

• Production output (as measured by the financial value or goods produced by employees) has increased by $35,000, so GP = $35,000.

• Employees' absenteeism caused by low-back injury declined 2%, resulting in a drop of $4,000, so PI = $4,000.

• The cumulative program intervention cost for operating the program is $35,000, so C = $35,000.

If we apply the preceding data to the net benefit equation, it is as follows:

Net benefit = [$90,000 + $35,000 + $4,000]
– $35,000 = $94,000

When one considers that the program has generated savings at almost three times its cost, the intervention clearly seems worth it.

Another common method used to econometrically evaluate WHP programs is the benefit-cost ratio (BCR), calculated by dividing the sum of all program-related benefits by the sum of all program costs. That is,

$$BCR = B/C$$

For example, consider a migraine headache control program that generated cost-avoidance savings of $50,000 through reduced migraine-related medical care and migraine-related absenteeism costs, compared to an annual intervention cost of $20,000:

$$B/C = \$50,000/\$20,000 = \$2.50/\$1.00$$

Note that the final step is to divide both the upper and lower figures by the lower number. This calculation will always result in $1.00 as the denominating unit of cost. Thus, in our example, a preliminary benefit-cost ratio of $50,000 to $20,000 would apply, and dividing both figures by $20,000 reveals that for every $1 of costs, benefits worth $2.50 were achieved. Evaluators can compare the preceding ratio to that of another program if they want to determine which of the two programs is most cost-effective. By doing so, a BCA can be used as a prerequisite for a cost-effectiveness analysis. For example, suppose the preceding program's benefit-cost ratio is compared with that of a low-back injury prevention program that yields the following ratio:

$$B/C = \$20,000/\$3,000 = \$6.66/\$1.00$$

Although both programs are successful, the low-back injury prevention program produced a better benefit-cost ratio, and from an econometric viewpoint, it is as important to the organization's financial welfare as the migraine control program.

## WHAT WOULD YOU DO?

Upon reviewing HRAs and health care claims data, you notice an increase in diabetes-related cases and costs compared to last year's experience. While preparing a proposal for a diabetes education and management program, you anticipate that your boss will ask you how the program will be evaluated and when the program will begin to pay off. What type of evaluation framework is most appropriate—a cost-effectiveness, a benefit-cost, or a break-even analysis? Which approach would you choose, and why?

# IV

# Managing Essential Worksite Health Promotion Considerations

# Overcoming Challenges of Company Size

After reading this chapter you will be able to

→ Identify several barriers that small businesses must overcome to establish successful WHP programs.

→ Describe how some small businesses pool their resources to provide employee health insurance.

→ Explain how a small business may use a "release time" staffing arrangement for WHP programming.

→ Compare the program planning process used in multisite settings versus a single worksite.

→ Distinguish between the scope of evaluating WHP programs in small, single-site settings and multisite settings.

Since 1985, three national surveys have been conducted to characterize and quantify health promotion awareness and activities in worksites with 50 or more employees. These studies consistently found that company size was a prominent indicator of the quantity and type of health promotion activities offered at the worksite. Worksites with over 750 employees consistently offered far more health promotion activities than smaller worksites; the smallest worksites in these studies, those with 50 to 99 employees, consistently offered fewer programs than the larger companies.

Although none of the preceding surveys included companies with fewer than 50 employees, findings from a 2001 survey of 2,000 small businesses—including those with fewer than 50 employees—indicated all of the following:

1. The most common health promotion activities are safety related (and therefore mandated by law).

2. The smallest businesses have less health promotion programming than larger ones.

3. The smallest businesses report higher participation rates than larger ones.

Overall, results from several surveys suggest that employees in small businesses are more likely to participate in health promotion programs than employees of larger businesses, but they have only limited access to them. Thus, most workers, being employed in small businesses, are an underserved population with regard to health promotion programming.

According to the U.S. Small Business Administration, small firms (those employing 2 to 500 people) represent 99% of all employers in the United States. The National Federation of Independent Businesses estimates that 60% of all businesses have fewer than four employees and 80% have fewer than 20 employees. And with the advent of downsizing, demographic shifts, and an expanding service sector, more employees find themselves working in smaller, decentralized (multisite) worksites. Moreover, many of these worksites are culturally diverse and may require different strategies from those of traditional WHP programs.

In this chapter we discuss the challenges involved in planning programs that are accessible and appropriate for employees at small, multisite, and culturally diverse worksites. Although these challenges are real, WHP professionals can almost always develop a sound and effective WHP strategy to suit a company's circumstances.

# SMALL BUSINESSES

Research shows that many small business owners are interested in WHP activities but feel they lack adequate resources to plan and implement them. Many of them cite the following obstacles to overcome in their quest to provide WHP:

- *Productivity demands.* Being preoccupied with productivity and cost issues, many small-business owners neglect human resource programs, including health promotion.
- *Poor financial support.* Small profit margins may limit funding for some programs.
- *No trained personnel.* Most small worksites lack human resource departments, safety coordinators, occupational health nurses, and WHP specialists who can oversee the development and provision of employee health promotion programs and services.
- *Lack of time.* Most small businesses operate with a minimum of workers in labor-intensive jobs with little or no flex-time.
- *Regulatory overkill.* Many small-business owners feel overwhelmed by occupational safety and health legislation and are often resistant to develop health-related programs not mandated by law.
- *Lack of facilities and equipment.* The initial expense of equipment and modifying part of the facility for fitness and health programs often makes small-business owners view WHP as a luxury they cannot afford.
- *Expectations of low participation.* Decision makers may think too few people would participate in WHP to justify the resources needed for a program to a captive audience.
- *Limited space.* Many small-business operations—service stations, convenience stores, fast food outlets—don't have adequate space to offer on-site programs.
- *Geographic dispersion.* Travel obligations of employees working in transportation, consulting, delivery, and sales positions limit their access to health promotion opportunities.
- *Multiple worksites.* Small numbers of employees working at several satellite locations are difficult to reach effectively with limited resources.

Despite these obstacles, small businesses have several advantages over large companies in planning worksite health promotion programs. For example, small businesses have fewer people to accommodate, which means less expense and less space to manage. Second, small businesses have more of a family-oriented and close-knit community than large corporations, promoting an environment that favors group participation. Third, local health agencies and organizations offering free or low-cost services often prefer to serve smaller companies. Finally, employee health improvements are more visible to coworkers in small worksites, thereby increasing the chance that others might be more motivated to participate.

## Health and Productivity Management

The explicit connection between health and productivity has spawned several relatively new WHP concepts of particular value to program planners and decision makers at all levels. For example, health and productivity management (HPM) operates on the belief that an at-risk workforce is a business risk with both direct and hidden costs that affect overall productivity. In fact, a growing body of literature is evolving to build the case that managing employee health is an essential, yet often overlooked, component of productivity management. In exploring this connection, consider that worksite health can improve a firm's overall productivity by

- attracting top-notch workers in a competitively global marketplace,
- reducing absenteeism and lost time,
- improving on-the-job decision making and use of time (reduced presenteeism),
- improving employee morale and fostering stronger organizational commitments,

- reducing management–labor conflicts by creating a heightened spirit of goodwill between key stakeholder groups, and
- reducing employee turnover.

The first step for a small business to achieve maximum health and productivity management benefits is to sponsor an affordable health care plan for employees. Most experts agree that WHP programs, when properly implemented, can help a small business achieve its health and productivity management goals, including health risk reduction and health care cost control. As many small-business owners can testify, strategies to contain their health care costs are particularly challenging when even one employee's poor health and medical misfortunes might significantly damage the bottom line. Although many small-business owners know the importance of having a good health insurance plan to protect against such risks, fewer than 50% of all small businesses actually provide basic health insurance coverage for their employees. It is ironic that nearly two thirds of persons without health insurance are in families headed by a full-time worker, most working at very small businesses. The high cost of providing health insurance coverage to employees and dependents is prohibitive for many small-business owners. Consequently, employees at these businesses are forced to personally shop the insurance market for the best deal, often changing insurers every year. Millions of others go without health insurance, forced to risk the devastating consequences of accidents or long-term illness because they simply cannot afford to pay rising health insurance premiums.

Some small companies are helping their employees obtain health insurance through health insurance pooling. A well-publicized example is a group of small businesses in Cleveland, Ohio, that formed a large pool called the Council of Smaller Enterprises (COSE). The council consists of nearly 17,000 member companies representing more than 225,000 covered employee lives throughout northeast Ohio. All COSE members can purchase affordable health insurance coverage because the Council has persuaded large insurers to offer their coalition the same advantages given to larger companies. The most important of these advantages is the clout to pressure doctors and hospitals to keep costs down. The COSE arrangement has been a successful cost-control strategy for its members,

whose annual premiums typically rise only about one fourth as much as those in non-COSE businesses. For more information on the Council, consult their Web site at www.cose.org. In addition, the Consumer Health Education Council (CHEC) provides a Web site portal of links to assist small-business owners in getting health insurance for their employees. The CHEC Web site is found at http://healthchec.org/employer/employer.html.

Increasingly, the availability and cost of a company's health care plan often depends on employees' health risks. In such a case, a company might only be able to afford insurance that does not pay claims directly tied to a person's choice, such as smoking-induced lung disease or injuries received during motor vehicle accidents in which safety belts were not worn. Or the company might be willing to pay the difference if their lifestyle choices result in higher risk. In either of these cases, a primary goal of WHP would be to motivate high-risk and unhealthy employees to reduce their risk factors.

## Planning

A greater understanding of existing health promotion programs in small businesses is critical if health professionals expect to increase the number of health promotion programs in these businesses. According to some experts, a key prerequisite for establishing a successful WHP in small business is management support. While some business owners strongly believe in employee health promotion programs, others are less enthusiastic and require evidence before they will support WHP efforts. When possible, consult with other WHP professionals in your community to learn why their small-business programs succeed (or why they have failed). For an example of a successful small-business program, see the profile on the Robert E. Mason Company on page 140.

To plan appropriate health promotion activities and programs, small businesses should follow the same procedures as larger businesses. The procedural guidelines tied to identification, assessment, planning, implementation, and evaluation (as discussed in chapters 2, 3, 5, and 6) are the same regardless of the size of a business. Yet, when you plug the unique characteristics of a small business into the general planning process, a proposal for WHP should be modified around these characteristics. For instance, WHP

## WHP on Release Time

The Robert E. Mason Company in Charlotte, North Carolina, has a workforce of about 100 employees. Two employees—the operations manager and the sales secretary—are given release time to administer the company's health promotion programs. Mason's operations manager states: "I am responsible for developing and implementing an administrative framework in which all of my official duties—including health insurance benefits and the after-work fitness program—are part of an integrated network of services" (see figure 9.1).

Whether the operations manager is involved in a personnel function such as doing a new-employee orientation or writing an article for the company's newsletter, she always thinks about ways to promote the company's commitment toward employee health. For instance, how can she integrate incentives in the benefits package to motivate all employees and dependents to promote their health? Although the impact of health promotion on employee health and overall cost-management goals is hard to measure, Mason has more employees participating in its health fair each year and more family members are becoming involved with the program.

Mason's WHP program has resulted in lower insurance costs. Insurance premium rate increases, directly tied to employee health claims, have decreased by as much as 5% in some years. Still, Mason has had to increase the employee deductible in some years, as well as raising each employee's out-of-pocket maximum in order to foster a culture of mutual employee–employer responsibility.

Mason's efforts have earned the company various statewide awards for its outstanding WHP programs.

planning for small business should provide for the following:

• *A flexible format.* For instance, WHP programs could be offered at the worksite or in a community center for several businesses to use collaboratively.

• *Simple equipment and space needs.* A small business does not need a large-scale exercise room or enough space to accommodate a large aerobics class. Modest arrangements for employees who want to improve their health are often enough to gain significant health increases among a small workforce.

• *Easy administration.* Again, nothing fancy is required. Programs that are relatively easy to plan and implement are often sufficient at smaller companies. For example, a prework low-back

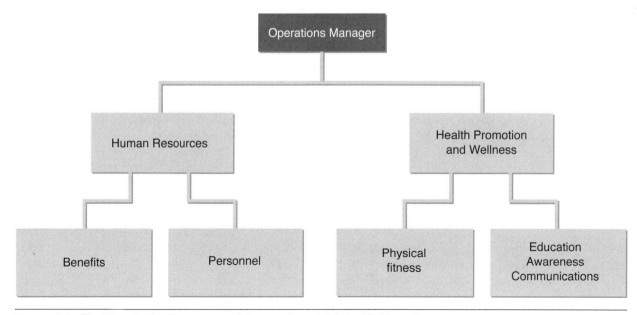

**Figure 9.1**   The integrated health management framework used at Robert E. Mason Company.
Courtesy of Robert E. Mason Company.

stretching and warm-up routine only requires a small area of open space and management support.

WHP programs do not have to be elaborate or expensive to be effective. In fact, most small worksite programs have no fitness facilities and require only a modest amount of money and time to administer the program. Many small businesses use community health agencies and vendors who can provide personnel, facilities, equipment, and instructional materials at little or no cost. Some of them work with the local chamber of commerce, local health departments, local merchants or trade associations, or shopping malls to hold events and activities. Some affordable small-scale options include the following:

• Sponsor on-site flu shots, blood pressure checks, diabetes screening, and so on. Check with your local health department; hospital; or nearby university health education, exercise science, and nursing departments to determine whether any of them can perform such services.

• Provide written materials such as self-care books, periodic newsletters, and a printed listing of Web sites that provide health-related news bits.

• Encourage and provide time for employees to exercise either before, during, or after work.

• Provide clean, safe, and accessible stairways to encourage stair climbing rather than using elevators or escalators.

• Offer financial incentives for employees who walk, ride a bike, take public transit, or carpool to work.

• Offer safe, secure, and free bike storage.

• Provide food choices in vending machines that meet healthy nutrition standards.

For additional employee health promotion strategies in small business, consult *Healthy Workforce 2010: An Essential Health Promotion Sourcebook for Employers, Large and Small,* published by Partnership for Prevention (www.prevent.org).

In some areas, small businesses can participate in community health alliances to offer WHP programs and activities to employees. For example, in north Texas, the Small Business Wellness Initiative is a community-collaborative project funded by a grant from the Department of Health and Human Services. The mission of the Initiative is to enhance the health, productiv-

ity, and quality of work life for small-business leaders, their employees, and their communities. Community partners include the Tarrant Council on Alcoholism & Drug Abuse, the North Texas Small Business Development Center, and Organizational Wellness & Learning Systems. For more information on the Initiative's model, programs, and services, access its Web site at www.sbwi.org.

Because most small businesses have a small (or nonexistent) budget for employee health promotion programs, employee volunteers or management might use an expense management grid (see chapter 5, page 71) as a guide to determine how to best use on-site and community resources. The grid can help a small business explore the feasibility of purchasing, renting, leasing, or brokering resources. For example, a rising percentage of small businesses are joining together with other small businesses to form pools to negotiate purchasing products and services at discounted rates. Services might include reduced employee membership fees at local health clubs, YMCAs, and community centers; affordable EAP services for local mental health clinics; and shared walking trails, school gymnasiums, parks, and athletic fields. Small-business health promoters should also carefully consider outsourcing.

Despite the growing success of small-business pools, many small companies might not have that option in their communities, so they must resort to one-to-one arrangements with local providers. If properly structured, these arrangements can benefit both parties. For instance, the partnership between the Wisconsin-based Copps grocery store chain and the YMCA has become a model for small businesses. Copps contracted with the Y to provide a three-phase WHP program consisting of fitness testing and consultation, health education, and special recreational opportunities. Nearly half of Copps' employees participate in the program. The success of the arrangement has had widespread value, benefiting not only Copps and the Y, but also the entire community as well other area businesses establish similar programs.

## Evaluation

Although they are not as likely as larger companies to have data-management systems for tracking absenteeism, productivity, health care use, and so on, small businesses can monitor certain types of data to evaluate their health promotion

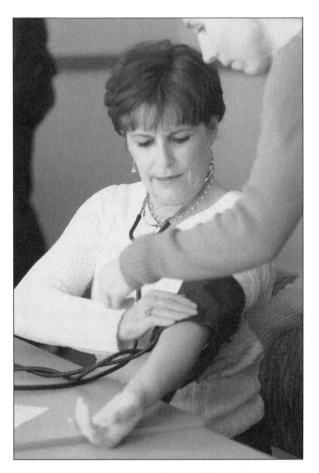

Staff and management can easily monitor health status indicators such as blood pressure, body fat percentage, and low-back flexibility to tell whether particular programs are working.

efforts. Chapter 8 discusses evaluation procedures that can be modified to suit small-business programs. At a minimum, employee participation should be tracked to evaluate interest in different types of health promotion programs.

In planning an evaluation, small businesses should not overlook possible assistance from local health associations and the prospects for creating collaborative arrangements. For example, faculty members at a local college may be interested in providing evaluation assistance in exchange for using a small worksite as a research site.

Although small businesses often need to find innovative ways to evaluate their programs, evaluation is a step that should never be neglected. A WHP program that is not evaluated cannot provide evidence that the program should be continued, greatly increasing the chances that management may consider WHP to be expendable.

Even relatively minor risk-reduction actions can pay off for small businesses. For example, consider two employees with chronic back problems: John works for a large company with 1,000 employees, whereas Michelle works for a small company with 20 employees. From a risk-management and economic point of view, John's health care costs associated with his back problem can be spread among 999 other employees, whereas Michelle's costs are spread among only 19 other employees. Consequently, on a per capita basis, Michelle's condition increases her company's health insurance risk 50 times more than John's condition, making it increasingly difficult for her company to qualify for—much less afford—today's costly health insurance coverage. Fortunately, today's health insurance pools (alliances) are closing this gap for many small businesses.

# MULTISITE SETTINGS

With trends continuing for businesses to place their workforces at multiple strategic or convenient locations, creating WHP programs to meet the needs of multisite companies has become a common challenge for health promoters. When working with multisite populations, WHP personnel will need to develop programs and policies based on the combined data from all sites. The data collected from site to site will often vary, and the program itself may need to vary in order to meet each site's unique needs. This tailoring is possible in large part because of the recent development of technology, mail-based initiatives, and online services that have opened up a lot of WHP options for small and multisite operations.

## Organizational Structure

Generally speaking, multisite businesses fall into two categories of organization: centralized, which is the traditional structure, and decentralized, a more contemporary structural organization. Refer to figures 9.2 and 9.3 for models of the two structures.

Multisite programming varies depending on the organizational structure. If a company is centralized, the headquarters facility generally funds and directs WHP programs to the field. The headquarters staff develops the materials and rolls out the program through field coordinators (who may or may not be health professionals). Although a company may be centralized and funded by corporate headquarters, if the local sites are dispersed throughout the country or abroad, cultural and demographic differences can greatly affect health promotion outcomes. In fact, even in a centralized operation it is not uncommon for headquarters to grant some autonomy for individual sites to tailor their WHP efforts around these unique characteristics.

If a company is decentralized, the local site tends to have more control over WHP programming. The local sites fund programs and generally want more customization. For example, a corporate health management goal may be to provide a safe and a healthy work environment. The operating division (individual site) may adapt this broad goal by adding specific goals, such as the following:

- Provide a back-injury prevention program to reduce back-injury costs by 50%.
- Provide healthy food options in the cafeteria.
- Encourage and help each employee achieve high levels of wellness and productivity.

Although a decentralized organization presents more challenges for WHP, a program director's considerations are similar for the two structures. In each case the director must find a way to modify the WHP planning framework (presented in the preface) to meet the needs of a multisite operation. In the sections that follow, the major components of the framework (identification, assessment, implementation, and evaluation) will be discussed as they relate to a company with employees spread among two or more locations.

## Identification and Assessment

As is true at a single-site location, planning WHP for a multisite program first involves identifying and assessing employee needs and interests. Thus, a health risk assessment is essential and should include biometric or clinical data to enhance the overall accuracy of these activities. Good assessment tools are particularly important to accurately gauge the prevalence of specific risk factors that warrant a clinical measurement rather than rely solely on self-report (e.g., obesity, hypertension, smoking, hyperlipidemia, and so on).

When a business has employees at several hard-to-reach or very different types of sites, identification and assessment become particularly important phases of the process. Review chapter 2 for details about these phases, and customize these activities around the unique characteristics and needs of your site. In particular, when conducting multisite programming, the key components within the two phases are to

- visit the sites and meet with management,
- learn current policies and procedures, and
- understand the site's operating systems (e.g., operations, databases, interdepartmental communication).

A first step is to visit the site and talk with key members of management. Depending on the number of locations, you may want to start with a survey to learn about employee demographics, areas of greatest need, shift schedules, cultural diversity, and types of work performed. You can mail this survey ahead of your visit so that you have time to weigh the results before you meet with employees and management.

To make your site visit more effective, talk to both management and employees to get an accurate perception of the operation. This is a good time to inquire about what types of community

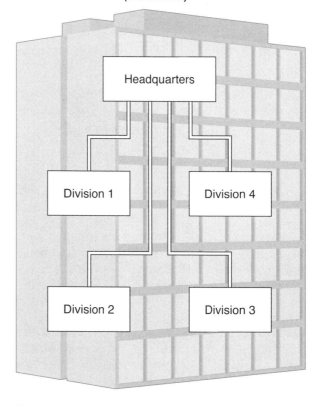

**Figure 9.2** A centralized (traditional) organizational structure.

**Decentralized Organization
(contemporary)**

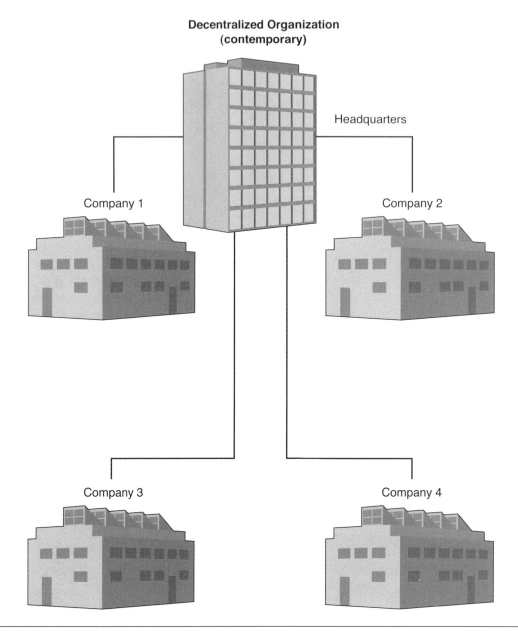

**Figure 9.3** A decentralized (contemporary) organizational structure.

health agencies and resources may be available in the area to assist small and multisite operations with their WHP efforts. Also, discuss safety issues, employee morale, common health problems seen in the workforce, health plan benefits, and whether union representation involved in employee health matters. If possible, see whether it's possible to observe and possibly work an off-schedule shift; this is a good opportunity to show employees that you are there to help them, not just management.

Along with meeting employees and management, inquire as to whether health care utiliza-

tion and cost data reports are available on-site. Such data may reveal specific types of health care services that are commonly used as well as types and locations of health care providers. This information may be particularly helpful when developing health care consumerism and self-care programs. Finally, try to meet with other human resources or WHP personnel at other worksites in the area to learn about their approach and experiences with employee health promotion.

During your site visit, get a copy of an employee handbook or policy and procedure manual. Review the document, looking at areas that influence the health of the work environment such as the site's smoking policy, flex-time policy, mandated safety or illness and injury prevention programs, sick leave and family leave, cafeteria and vending machine options, worksite violence prevention programs, drug screening programs, return-to-work programs, preemployment screening process, and other items relevant to employee health.

Understanding a site's operating systems allows for more comprehensive WHP planning to occur. The better you develop your programs to align with current organizational systems, the more likely the programs will be accepted and successful. During your site visit, talk to human resources or benefits personnel to learn how policies are monitored and modified, when necessary. If an employee union exists, also try to understand the union–management relationship and the process used to reach consensus. Other operating systems to inquire about include safety practices, medical management, communication systems, hiring and training practices, and total quality management practices. For example, when you offer on-site or online programming , if you don't have good systems in place with sound protocols for delivering the services, the quality of your programs may be jeopardized.

## Implementation

Refer to chapter 7 to review general guidelines for implementing WHP programs. In general, it pays to standardize the way you are implementing the programs in order to create a "turnkey" operation. Doing so will allow the person(s) in charge of implementing WHP activities to easily adopt and implement WHP activities. Additional steps involved in implementing programs specifically for multisite businesses include recruiting volunteer coordinators; considering the addition of staff to reach all sites; rewriting internal policies and procedures; following up on communication with management, employees, volunteers, and any WHP staff; developing programs to encourage self-responsibility; considering readiness to change; targeting high-risk employees; emphasizing self-care programs; and weighing other critical considerations. Each of these steps will be discussed in detail in the following section.

With limited resources, many multisite WHP programs are run by employee volunteers who have some release time from their official job duties to direct or provide such efforts. By and large, volunteers should

- be good role models,
- be respected by their peers,
- possess leadership and facilitative skills, and
- have a respect of and appreciation for employees' diversity (values, beliefs, lifestyles, and so on).

In the event that a committee of employee volunteers is responsible for directing or staffing WHP activities, it may be useful to develop a charter that can be used to guide and monitor personnel activities; it may include length of membership on the committee, roles and responsibilities, and expectations of communicating between and among various parties. In addition, volunteer committees will need ongoing support and guidance from a qualified and respected individual(s) to ensure responsibility and focus. Possible options may include assistance from the following:

- Local health department personnel skilled in WHP issues
- Local university faculty experienced in WHP issues
- WHP-savvy representatives from your health plan
- Outside WHP vendor who provides feedback and ideas at regular intervals

During the development and implementation of awareness and basic education programs for employees, a non-health professional can roll out and follow up with many program materials provided by you. But as the site matures and more focused education and behavior change programs are developed and implemented, the need for professional assistance arises. Staffing options vary depending on site funding and demand. Some of these options include the following:

- Providing internships for qualified students from a local university
- Hiring a local vendor skilled in WHP issues
- Hiring and training a local team of professionals to go on site-specific assignments
- Teaming with your current health plan to provide services at a reduced rate

Whatever options are used for staffing, it is important for all staff members to have a clear understanding of corporate-wide WHP goals and how site-specific WHP goals relate to the big picture. For example, provide all on-site staff with any customer research data and the marketing processes to make sure they understand management's view and level of commitment so that they can accommodate employees with disabilities and possible liability concerns. The better they fit into the cultural norms, the fewer barriers will exist to compromise participation.

For WHP programs to work in multisite settings, it is critical for company policies and program interventions to be properly aligned. For instance, smoking policies should support smoking cessation efforts, the cafeteria or vending machines should provide healthy meals consistent with existing nutrition and weight management programs, employee hours need to be flexible enough to allow participation in health promotion activities, and so on. Worksite health programs that are inconsistent with overall company policies reduce the programs' credibility and practically ensure failure.

Before implementing a program, revisit the initial discussions you had with site management to ensure that the program's goals match up with management expectations.

You might put agreements in writing to reconfirm all parties' commitment to responsibilities, costs, time lines, and follow-up procedures. The more health promotion is integrated with other company functions, the greater the importance of this communication, because all parties should be involved on a regular basis. This is particularly true because an individual WHP professional will not have a full-time presence in all sites of a multisite arrangement. Moreover, official job duties of WHP volunteers generally do not include health promotion responsibilities. Thus, it is simply not enough for WHP personnel to have an on-site presence; it is also important to make sure you have a good communications plan in place so that employees consistently understand who is responsible for conducting WHP activities at each site.

Many multisite programs do not have the benefit of having an on-site, full-time WHP specialist or health care professional. Although all programs should encourage employee self-responsibility, multisite populations without immediate resources need to be developed and implemented with self-responsibility in mind. Therefore, it's important to plan programs with a facilitative approach rather than a direct approach. Instead of telling employees what to do to be healthy, motivate them through education about the effects of their lifestyle choices. Give them options they can tailor to meet their goals and fit their situations and values. As one program director once put it, "We need to adopt the attitude that we may be great coaches, but we cannot ourselves get out there and win the ball game."

In dispersed workforces, organizational change and issues will be different. For example, one site may be in union negotiations, another may be downsizing, and still another may be undergoing a safety audit. Given the changing variables within each organization, program implementation may look different, and timing will vary from year to year on site requests. To ensure that organizational needs are met, develop core content that can be flexible and customized to cultural demands. When assessing individual need and readiness to change, factor in physiological risk factors, current behavior and habits, psychological factors, and social support. Most health risk appraisals provide this type of individual assessment. In addition, take the time to research and understand cultural predispositions to certain genetic health risks, as well as cultural lifestyle patterns. At this point an insightful occupational health nurse or human resources manager can shed some light on how a workforce's demographic, cultural, and lifestyle characteristics may influence employees' willingness to participate in your WHP programs. While tapping these insights, it's important to consider what can be done to assess where employees currently exist on the readiness-to-change continuum. This is a good time to consider DiClemente and Proschaska's stages of change:

1. **Precontemplation:** Individual is unaware, unwilling, or discouraged when changing problem behavior.

2. **Contemplation:** Individual is considering the prospects of change and researching information about the pros and cons of the change.

3. **Preparation:** Individual intends to make change in the near future; he or she has learned valuable lessons from past attempts and failures.

4. **Action:** Individual takes action to change behavior.

5. **Maintenance:** Individual attempts to sustain change and avoid relapse.

By assessing and gathering baseline data on individuals, you can better develop and implement different intervention options that will appeal to people at their personal level of readiness to change. In particular, explore your options to provide self-responsible options and choices from group programs to individual programs and from corporate-based models to community or health plan–based programs. Understand the culture to know whether tangible incentives extrinsically motivate employees to start behavior change. Thus, it's important to consult your volunteer committee members and local resources to enhance your programming decisions. Many times you will perceive an individual's readiness to change, but the worksite environment or cultural norms cannot support the process. At this point is where flexibility and knowledge as well as utilization of resources become critical.

It's important to further implementation efforts for multisite programs to encourage ongoing awareness campaigns, health fairs, and group education programs. While resources remain limited, shifting delivery from untargeted, group-based health promotion to targeting at-risk employees is proving to be a very cost-effective approach. To make the most impact, consider targeting the at-risk group that is the most ready to change.

Historically, WHP efforts have not adequately addressed relapse, which is the greatest barrier to permanent lifestyle change. Research conducted by StayWell Health Management Systems, Inc. indicated that targeting employees with high-risk profiles who are ready to change increases the potential for long-term behavior change (Anderson, 2003). High-risk employees generally require proactive, ongoing support. Note the comparison in table 9.1 of the traditional model versus the focused intervention model. Thus, by

**Table 9.1　A Comparison Between a Traditional and a Focused HPI**

| Traditional | Focused intervention |
| --- | --- |
| *General promotion* | *Personalized promotion* |
| Posters and flyers | Individualized based on interest, need, risk, and readiness |
| Newsletter articles | Target marketing to specific individuals |
| *Time-based assessment* | *Participation and risk-based assessment* |
| Annual or scheduled assessments | Targeting nonparticipants |
| | Individuals with specific risks would increase assessments |
| Not based on risk, just age and sex | New preventive exam schedules to focus on risk with follow-up appropriate to risk |
| *Untargeted group education* | *Individually focused education* |
| Same class to all; does not consider need or interest | Invitation to specific risk-based class |
| | Target to match individual need with type of education and individual preference |
| | Traditional class with group program but also offer one-on-one counseling or self-study |
| *Reactive maintenance* | *Proactive support and follow-up* |
| Problem of relapse is ignored or addressed only when relapse has occurred | Identify and build in support, counseling, and one-on-one opportunities as part of the delivery process |
| | Built-in maintenance, appropriate follow-up, and facilitation skills |
| *"Add-on" evaluation* | *Integrated evaluation* |
| Unfocused metrics | Built in to process prior to delivery |
| After-the-fact evaluation | Appropriate and effective measures focused on risk reduction |

Reprinted by permission from StayWell Health Management Systems, Inc.

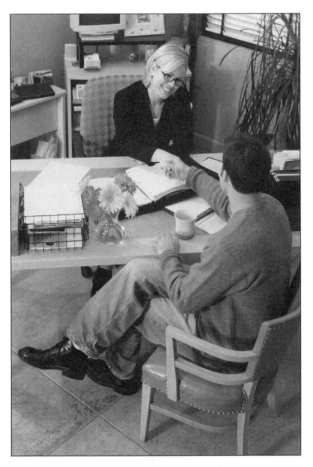

Focused interventions are designed specifically to identify and motivate high-risk individuals toward risk-reduction action.

shifting funds from group-based programming to a high-risk focus, you are more likely to impact your program goals sooner and sustain long-term results. Yet, in every worksite setting, it is important to provide WHP opportunities to all employees, including those classified as being at low risk. In fact, some research shows that it may be just as important to keep low-risk employees at low risk as it is to move high-risk employees to moderate- or low-risk status.

Medical self-care programs assist in lowering the demand for health care by helping employees enhance their decision-making skills, improve the quality of self-care they practice, and communicate effectively with their health care providers. In multisite work settings, it is not uncommon for employers to provide multiple employee health plans ranging from the traditional (and most expensive) indemnity, fee-for-service plan to today's managed care plans (e.g., HMO, PPO, POS, EPO). Because these plans vary widely in the number and type of health care providers,

benefit offerings, and the quality of customer service, it is vital for employees to learn how to navigate this maze of health care options as well as know when and how to assume personal responsibilities for minor aches and pains. With the advent of medical self-care and consumerism growing yearly, some companies are reporting benefit-cost ratios of 3:1 or better with such initiatives.

Multisite programs differ most in the need for flexibility and creativity in implementation and delivery methods. Factors such as decentralization, site-driven funding, culturally and occupationally diverse employee groups, limited staffing, organizational readiness, and individual readiness challenge the health professional to meet these multifaceted needs at different times and in customized ways. Niche programming for the local culture is critical. Spending time in their environment, especially with blue-collar employees, cultivates trust and a relevant understanding of their jobs, which is extremely important.

## Evaluation

Considerations for multisite program evaluation are often more complex than a single-site evaluation. Some issues unique to multisite evaluation are discussed in the following sections.

Throughout the life of the program, management support is essential. The more decentralized the program, the more time you find yourself spending to obtain ongoing support and focus for the health promotion program. It is wise to have a broad base of management support and not rely on one champion at the site. For example, you may have 40 sites, with five to seven managers at each site. The possibility for turnover and rotation of these managers creates an ongoing process of educating management on key issues, focus, and outcomes.

During the initial proposal writing and planning meeting with management, bring an evaluation plan to base decisions on. Managers who are unaware of the benefits of health promotion and preventive health services may have a difficult time in determining and articulating their desired outcome. Lead them by offering options, especially in a multisite environment where decentralized managers are looking for specific goals. An effective and cost-efficient strategy is to facilitate consensus of goals and objectives across all multisite management teams. Work with the

# Preventive Health Services Management Satisfaction Survey

Thank you in advance for sharing your input on Preventive Health Services (PHS). Your response is very important to our continuous improvement process. Because we are requesting feedback from several different perspectives at many of Chevron's worksites, we would greatly appreciate it if you would complete this survey yourself and not pass it on to someone else. Please return this survey by October 12th to the address on the reverse side.

## I. Each statement below describes a specific aspect of Preventive Health Services (PHS).

Using the following scale, please indicate how much you agree or disagree with each statement.

| Strongly disagree | Disagree | Somewhat disagree | Somewhat agree | Agree | Strongly agree |
|---|---|---|---|---|---|

1. Our PHS advisor has contacted me to describe the range of services PHS provides.

   1      2      3      4      5      6

2. PHS is an important resource because it helps my employees be more productive.

   1      2      3      4      5      6

3. PHS provides information that helps create and maintain a healthy workforce in order to meet our business objectives.

   1      2      3      4      5      6

4. My employees utilize PHS.

   1      2      3      4      5      6

5. Our PHS advisor responds to our needs quickly.

   1      2      3      4      5      6

6. Our PHS advisor sees goals and priorities to accomplish results.

   1      2      3      4      5      6

7. Our PHS advisor demonstrates the expertise to meet our needs.

   1      2      3      4      5      6

8. Our PHS advisor suggests creative solutions to address our needs.

   1      2      3      4      5      6

9. Our PHS advisor works effectively with us or our employees to deliver services.

   1      2      3      4      5      6

10. Our PHS advisor expresses her-/himself clearly.

    1      2      3      4      5      6

11. Our PHS advisor demonstrates effective presentation skills.

    1      2      3      4      5      6

12. Our PHS advisor gives us a written annual summary of services delivered.

    1      2      3      4      5      6

13. The services offered by PHS have been of benefit to my employees in areas such as employee safety, health, and commitment to the company and are therefore worth the cost.

    1      2      3      4      5      6

14. I will continue to use PHS.

    1      2      3      4      5      6

*(continued)*

## II. We have used the following PHS (check all that apply):

☐ Annual wellness program

☐ Back-injury prevention

☐ ERT/firefighter physical conditioning

☐ Fitness facility consultation

☐ Health education

☐ Health fair

☐ Health plan coordination (regarding preventive services)

☐ Health risk assessment and blood pressure or cholesterol screening

☐ Health Quest University

☐ Healthy cafeteria/vending nutritional consultation

☐ Initial PHS consultation

☐ Newsletter/health awareness articles

☐ Office ergonomics

☐ Smoking policy development and smoking cessation programs

☐ Other: _____

## III. My primary reasons for utilizing PHS are (rank the following reasons with 1 as the most important) as follows:

☐ Demonstrate commitment to employees and their health.

☐ Improve on/off job safety.

☐ Increase employee morale.

☐ Increase employee productivity.

☐ Reduce health-related risks.

☐ Support incident-free operations.

☐ Other: _____

## IV. Please tell us something about yourself.

Your work type:     ☐ Human resources     ☐ Safety     ☐ Other _____

## V. COMMENTS:

_____

_____

_____

_____

_____

Courtesy of Chevron Preventive Health Services.

organization's business plan and metrics and lay out the evaluation plan within the existing framework. Be realistic in your evaluation plan; use multisite reporting in the data, writing the data parameters you need from each site in order to meet its goals and objectives. For example, you need either to receive health plan utilization from human resources or you need a copy of the monthly incident report. Reach a consensus with other functional groups on how this data should look when you receive this information.

Program tracking is the most critical component of a multisite program and evaluation. The need for a data-management system and clear utilization process to link the integrated program is key to evaluation success. Linking systems through a computer wide area network, local area network, integrated health data management systems (IHDMS), or e-mail to coordinate the multisite data collection are good options. For very small multisite locations, a strategy may be to have WHP staff complete a standard evaluation form to send to a centralized data collection site. In any case, the tracking system for evaluation must be clearly thought out, planned, and funded at the outset of the program.

Program effectiveness is usually gauged by the ratio of benefit to cost. With multisite programs, you may be required to report by location. Suppose one of your multiple sites decides to implement a program that includes an initial survey, a health fair with HRAs and screenings, and a high-risk targeted follow-up for 10% of the site employees. How will you measure this one site's return on investment? Does the benefit-cost ratio fit your overall strategy to support the goals and objectives? Or, given the scope of your programs, is it more practical to simply track changes in participation or risk-factor status?

The data-tracking system should enable seamless recording of participation levels. Be prepared to measure specific types of participation based on utilization, penetration, and adherence rates. At a minimum, the number of employees in attendance should be tracked, and utilization and penetration should be readily available, if requested. Each independent site should be given feedback as well as aggregate data collected on all multiple sites. It is customary to monitor employee adherence to an activity and track behavior change. It may also be valuable to record how many high-risk employees attended the program and improved.

Planning processes are essential to ensure consistent development and growth of your program. As integration at each multisite heightens, the more checks and balances are needed to ensure process efficiency. Process evaluation of each functional group and the integration links are critical to maximizing outcomes and program impact. Other functional groups collect data in collaboration with a data-management system or independently (e.g., health plan utilization, safety records, and workers' compensation data). Yet the overall process of data integration impacts outcomes. The opportunity for duplication of services, costs, and low communication grows as the integration spreads without control.

Survey your multisite management customers throughout the life of the program to ensure site-specific satisfaction and to then gather feedback. Distribution of an employee survey measuring the level of commitment, behavior-change opinions, assessing motivational levels, and providing the opportunity to offer feedback allow refocus and insurance for program impact. An important goal of an evaluation strategy is to provide

## Table 9.2 Listing and Description of WHP Services Offered by Chevron's PHS to Chevron Worksites Worldwide

| WHP Services | Description |
|---|---|
| PLANNING/ASSESSMENT | |
| Annual plan | A PHS advisor discusses your business needs and describes PHS services available. A plan is made jointly by the PHS advisor and on-site staff for the delivery of specific services that involve outside vendors. |
| Health plan coordination | Work with Chevron health plans to evaluate preventive services and maximize their accessibility to their employees and their families; often includes free delivery of health promotion services at the worksite. |

*(continued)*

Table 9.2   (continued)

| WHP Services | Description |
|---|---|
| **HEALTH RISK ASSESSMENT (HRA)** | |
| Blood pressure/cholesterol screening | Provide an HRA, which uses medical screening values (blood pressure and cholesterol) and a health questionnaire to identify employee health risks. All employees receive feedback. Groups with 50+ HRAs completed receive an aggregate report of group risks. Repeat HRAs every 3 years and screenings annually. |
| Initial consult | Review PHS business plan and cost/services. Discuss customer needs and business values. |
| **AWARENESS** | |
| Health fair | Coordinate an event during which health-related vendors provide materials on a variety of health and wellness topics for the purpose of increasing participant awareness of health issues and referral sources. Vendors usually include Chevron health plans. |
| Health Quest University | Provide turnkey modules on health promotion topics that address health risk areas. Topics include back injury prevention, shift work, and nutrition. Ideal for safety meetings. |
| Newsletter articles | Develop and distribute schedules of services and programs or articles within local newsletters focusing on healthy lifestyle topics. PHS provides articles on a wide range of topics. |
| Preventive exam | Coordinate an annual or biannual reminder to all employees on their birthdays, encouraging them to schedule a preventive exam and explaining the guidelines for preventive exam content. |
| **HEALTHY WORKPLACE** | |
| Fitness center | Provide guidance on establishing supervised or unsupervised facilities with aerobic programs and cardiovascular, strength, and endurance equipment. Facilities offer a variety of health and fitness programs to encourage healthy lifestyle habits. |
| Healthy cafeteria/vending and nutritional consultation | Provide suggestions to caterers regarding healthy choices and alternatives in menu selections. Work with customers on providing healthy choices in the vending machines. |
| Smoking control policy | Written smoking cessation policy exists and is communicated at the site. |
| Back health | Train supervisors, employees, and ergonomics committees to review correct lifting mechanics, apply NIOSH guidelines to work situations, and address behavior change to prevent injury. |
| ERT/firefighter physical conditioning | Train ERT and firefighters including a physical assessment and exercise guidelines applicable to ERT duties, safe lifting, and back injury prevention. |
| Office ergonomics | Train supervisors, employees, and employee coaches to identify correct ergonomic principles and encourage behavior change to prevent injury. |
| Pretask safety stretching | Implementation of a stretching program prior to work and/or doing physical tasks, in an effort to reduce potential injury. |
| **BEHAVIOR CHANGE** | |
| Nutrition and weight control | Provide guidance to work groups on healthy eating (i.e., control room cooking classes and/or weight management programs). |
| **INCENTIVE PROGRAM** | |
| Consultation/development | Provide guidance on effective, appropriate incentives to motivate all employees to participate in healthy lifestyle activity. |
| Medical self-care and health care consumerism | A comprehensive medical self-care book is made available to all employees. Use of the book is reinforced through training and incentives. |
| Smoking control | Employees are aware that smoking cessation resources are readily available. Resources are varied and range from self-help materials to referral to group programs. |

Courtesy of Chevron Preventive Health Services.

feedback that you will continually communicate to management and employees.

Multisite program planning requires consistent communication, clarification, and follow-up to management customers. Organizations in continually changing environments have a tendency to work as a single site in a vacuum, which creates barriers for the programmer planning multisite global processes. Critical success factors for a multisite program manager include high integration, along with reaching all levels of employees with communications and program penetration. Ensure this by working with them on their shift, in their work environment; be real and honest with these employees. Ask the customer what is wrong with the program and how it can be improved. Customers are your ultimate audience, and their empowering trust to you only comes with real personal presence and experience.

## WHAT WOULD YOU DO?

In your quest to find a summer job, you land a part-time sales position with a small auto parts distributor (50 employees). During your first week, the human resources director distributes a storewide memo (a) announcing that the store's health care costs have increased 25% over the past year, (b) that nearly 50% of the increased costs are caused by low-back injury claims, and (c) that all employees will have to contribute $150 more per month to maintain their health insurance benefits. As you size up the situation, the thought of proposing a prework low-back stretching program on work time comes to mind. You assume that such a program (a) may demonstrate to the health insurer that the store is committed to reducing its low-back injury risk and (b) would buy more time for the store to show that it can lower this risk and associated costs. With your game plan in mind, what obstacles should you consider in selling this proposal to the human resources director and eventually to the insurer to give the program a chance to reduce low-back risks?

---

Read the following descriptions of different worksites, all of which are part of the same corporation, and choose one.

• **Case study 1:** A coal mine in New Mexico employs 85% Navajo American Indians. Total employee population is 375 people (90% men and 10% women). The mine is unionized and works three rotating 8-hour shifts. The mine has three different sites with separate entrances. The union participates in a nationwide health plan negotiated specifically for coal miners, which includes little preventive care. Management will only participate and pay for preventive activities if employees drive the program.

• **Case study 2:** A refinery employs 90% men and 10% women. The total employee population is 1,200, with an average age of 42. The nonunion workforce requires 70% heavy labor done in two rotating 12-hour shifts. A health promotion program has been in place for 2 years with an on-site fitness facility of 10,000 square feet. The top employee risk factors are poor eating habits, stress, back injuries, high blood cholesterol, and lack of daily aerobic exercise.

• **Case study 3:** In a large midwestern city, a cellular phone company has five worksites with a total of 1,500 white-collar employees. The population is 50% male and 50% female, and the average employee age is 34. The majority of employees have a college education, and the company is nonunion. Access to health promotion and risk-reduction programs is limited to the choice of two managed care programs.

• **Case study 4:** Located on the East Coast are 55 offshore oil platforms, which house 15 to 40 employees at each bunkhouse. Each facility has a catered food arrangement and 17 have functioning fitness facilities. The population is nonunion and 90% blue-collar males. The employees belong to a traditional indemnity (fee-for-service) plan and emergency care is the most common claim.

After reviewing the strategies for multisite WHP programs described in this chapter, select one of the case study sites and create ideas for conducting each of the four activities listed below:

1. Employee research (needs and interest)
2. Marketing
3. Development and implementation
4. Evaluation

# Beginning a Successful Career

After reading this chapter you will be able to

→ Identify several WHP skills most highly preferred by prospective employers.

→ Describe how certification and professional resources can enhance your professional preparation.

→ List several factors to consider in preparing for a WHP internship.

→ Demonstrate good interviewing skills in a mock interview.

**W**HP programs in American worksites grew at an unprecedented rate from the early 1970s until the late 1990s. However, in the past decade, the WHP program growth has slowed, in part because of economic, political, and financial factors. While some industry watchers predict a continuation of little or no growth into the next decade, others view WHP as an essential business strategy for workforces to stay competitive in today's global economy. What does the future have in store for WHP programs and aspiring professionals? This question is certainly provocative and timely, considering the turbulent economic times we live in. However, given today's increased emphasis on health and productivity management at many worksites, this field has a promising future, especially for enthusiastic and energetic individuals who prepare for it.

What are the essential skills for successfully entering today's competitive job market? According to two independent surveys—one involving nearly 200 WHP program directors from educational, corporate, and hospital settings—certain behaviors, knowledge, and skills are highly desirable (see the following lists). Overall, the surveys reflect an increased emphasis on a broad

| Behaviors | Knowledge areas | Skills |
|---|---|---|
| Shows initiative | Behavior change | Motivating participants |
| Models healthy lifestyle | Physical health | Presentations |
| Demonstrates teamwork | Stress management | Assessing fitness |
| Is sensitive to diversity | Nutrition | Health counseling |
| Does more than job requires | Aerobic exercise | Assess and interpret health data |
| Respects company policies | Emotional health | Marketing |
| Knows and uses clients' names | Health care utilization | Leading behavior change groups |
| | Health care costs | |
| | Using health care data for programs | |
| | Designing incentive programs | |
| | Evaluating programs | |

background, especially for those hoping to become program managers or directors (Rojas-Guyler, Cottrell, and Wagner, 2006; Jones and Ver Voort, 1995).

# ACADEMIC PREPARATION

To meet the growing health management needs of many employers, various universities offer courses and degrees in WHP and related disciplines. Because academic programs typically reflect the philosophies of their faculty, it is important for aspiring WHP professionals to compare curricula closely before enrolling in a particular program. Ask to see copies of course syllabi so that you can evaluate the topics covered in each course. Review this information and talk with a faculty member to determine whether a particular academic program really reflects today's marketplace and your career interests.

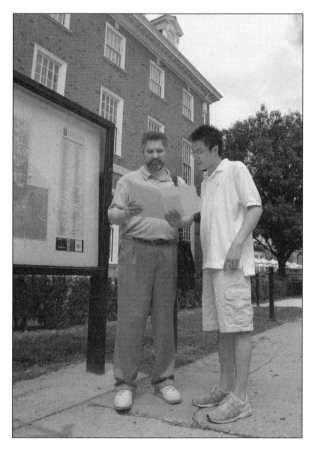

Take the time to speak with faculty members to learn about a program's curriculum, faculty experience in the field of WHP, internship opportunities, where past graduates are working, graduate school possibilities, and job prospects after graduation.

If possible, select a program that has a strong foundation in health promotion that can be complemented with courses in exercise science, business management, and any other ancillary area in which an academic minor or specific certification is sought. Overall, a good academic program should provide you with a true perspective of what is happening in the WHP area locally, regionally, and nationally as well as practical or internship exposure in a real worksite setting.

To succeed in today's competitive marketplace, you need a strong base of skills in health promotion, exercise science, and business management. A multifaceted background is particularly important; career options evolve, and companies look for one person to serve multiple roles. Having a versatile background can also be the crucial ingredient for moving into advanced positions.

## Developing a Competitive Academic Program

In preparing for a successful career in WHP, work closely with your academic advisor to develop a competitive academic program that makes full use of your elective hours. For example, avoid filling these elective hours with easy courses just to boost your GPA because a handful of soft A's won't win you many points in the job market. Today's marketplace is increasingly competitive, so prepare for your future by making your curriculum competitive, too. The following are among the upper-level courses you should consider taking:

| | |
|---|---|
| Anatomy and physiology | Business management |
| Health behavior | Business speech |
| Health problems | Human nutrition |
| Injury/accident control | Business law |
| Exercise physiology | Management |
| Exercise testing and prescription | Industrial psychology |
| | Marketing |
| Exercise instruction | Risk management |
| Program planning | Accounting |
| Program evaluation | Stress management |
| First aid and CPR | Medical terminology |

To further enhance your job prospects, seriously consider a minor in business administration, occupational safety, allied health, or another area related to WHP. In keeping abreast of the ever-changing nature of today's worksite climate, learn as much as you can about as many things as you can. Read widely from health promotion, fitness, and business publications to keep apprised of today's key issues and trends in WHP.

During your senior year, talk to your academic advisor to learn more about certification opportunities, professional conferences, and internship opportunities. Also, be sure to sign up with your university's job placement (career) center. Many university job placement centers sponsor workshops to assist students in writing application letters, creating effective resumes, and successfully interviewing with a prospective employer.

## Certification

Over the past two decades, the percentage of WHP-related job descriptions that require one or more types of certification has substantially increased. Thus, it is important for your academic program to provide the right type of knowledge and skills for you to qualify for appropriate certifications. For example, if you are pursuing a university program in quest for a particular certification, ask the faculty or your advisor the following questions:

- Which courses will help me prepare for specific certifications relevant to my chosen occupation?

- When is the best time to take these courses—independently, in combination, in my senior year, or just prior to an internship?

- Is a study group or other preinternship exam activity available to help me prepare for a certification exam?

- Does the university sponsor any on-site certification exams throughout the academic year? If not, what is the closest university offering these exams?

- How desirable are specific certifications in the marketplace?

- What distinguishes one certification from another?

- Once a person earns a particular certification, is an ongoing program (such as continuing education) available to help the person remain certified?

Table 10.1 provides a listing of various certification programs for WHP and fitness specialists.

## Professional Publications and Conferences

A good way to learn about and stay apprised of the latest WHP research and trends is to access

### Table 10.1 Selected Certifications for WHP and Fitness Specialists

| Organization | Web site address | Certifications |
| --- | --- | --- |
| Aerobics and Fitness Association of America (AFAA) | www.afaa.com | Group Exercise, Kickboxing, Yoga, Personal Training, Pilates, and others |
| American College of Sports Medicine (ACSM) | www.acsm.org | Health/Fitness Instructor, Exercise Specialist, Registered Clinical Physiologist, Certified Personal Trainer, Health/Fitness Instructor, and Exercise Specialist |
| American Council on Exercise (ACE) | www.acefitness.org | Personal Training, Group Fitness Instructor, Lifestyle and Weight Management Consultant, and others |
| American Lung Association | www.lungusa.com | Freedom from Smoking Facilitator |
| The Cooper Institute | www.cooperinst.org | Fitness Specialist, Group Exercise, Pre-/Postnatal Fitness, and others |
| The National Commission for Health Education Credentialing, Inc. (NCHEC) | www.nchec.org | Certified Health Educator Specialist (CHES) |
| National Strength and Conditioning Association (NSCA) | www.nsca-cc.org | NSCA Certified Personal Trainer |

various professional journals and publications. Many journals have abstracts of selected articles that you can access free of charge at their respective Web sites; full articles are available to paying subscribers. Some publishers provide student membership discounts on their publications. A listing of WHP related publications is shown in table 10.2.

Most of the listed organizations also sponsor conferences that provide excellent opportunities for attendees to learn about the latest events, network with others, and explore internship and job opportunities.

## The University Affiliate Program

A valuable resource for universities preparing WHP practitioners is the University Affiliate Program (UAP), which is created and administered by Wellness Councils of America (WELCOA). UAP is an initiative designed to strengthen and enhance health promotion curricula of participating colleges and universities by providing them with the latest WHP information. Colleges and universities taking part in the UAP are given a complimentary subscription to WELCOA's *Absolute Advantage* magazine and InfoPoint Web site. Both of these resources are currently utilized by over 2,500 corporate members as points of reference for worksite health promotion. Published 10 times a year, *Absolute Advantage* includes tips and strategies, unique insights, and real-life studies from some of the best WHP programs in the country. InfoPoint is home to several resources that are of great value to both students and health promotion professionals alike. Additional areas of interest available at the InfoPoint Web site include archives (past issues) of *Absolute Advantage*, how-to guides, downloadable presentations, case studies, a wellness library, and career center. Colleges and universities interested in becoming UAP members should e-mail their requests to wellworkplace@welcoa.org.

### Table 10.2 Professional Publications and Web Listings

| Publication | Web site contact |
|---|---|
| *WELCOA's Absolute Advantage* | www.welcoa.org |
| *ACSM's Health & Fitness Journal* | www.acsm.org |
| *American Journal of Health Studies* | http://ajhs.tamu.edu/ |
| *American Journal of Health Promotion* | www.healthpromotionjournal.com |
| *Employer Health Management eNews* | www.thebenfieldgroup.com |
| *Health & Productivity Management* | www.ihpm.org |
| *Health Promotion Practitioner* | www.nationalwellness.org |
| *HERO e-newsletter* | www.the-hero.org |
| *IDEA Fitness Journal* | www.ideafit.com |
| *IDEA Trainer Success* | www.ideafit.com |
| *IDEA Fitness Manager* | www.ideafit.com |
| *American Association of Occupational Health Nursing Journal* | www.aaohn.org |
| *Journal of Physical Activity and Health* | www.HumanKinetics.com |
| *Journal of Occupational and Environmental Medicine* | www.acoem.com |
| *Occupational Health & Safety* | www.stevenspublishing.com |
| *Platinum Book: Health & Productivity Management* | www.ihpm.org |
| *Measuring Employee Productivity* | www.ihpm.org |
| *The Physician and Sportsmedicine* | www.acsm.org |
| *Wellness Management* | www.nationalwellness.org |

# Internships

One of the best ways to enhance your marketability is to have some worksite experience before entering the job market. Many business, industrial, governmental, military, and health care organizations offer internships, which can provide valuable experience in developing and refining your skills in an actual worksite. One student summed up his internship this way:

> This internship has been a wonderful learning experience for me. It showed me that I could interact with a wide array of people and help them meet their special needs. I also benefited from my exposure to the employee health screenings that I would not have gotten through the university. This experience helped hone my writing skills. This internship has made me more self-reliant (in part because of my newly-developed computing skills) and increased my self-confidence. I have recognized my shortcomings, too—frustration at setbacks and the need to prepare further in advance. Overall, this internship was a period of tremendous growth, both professionally and personally. This is the result of the staff carefully preparing our activities for the summer by the entire staff. A contributing factor to my growth was the amount of "hands-on" experience we (student interns) received.

If you are interested in doing an internship, meet with your academic advisor to discuss internship opportunities related to your career interest. Because intern responsibilities and employer expectations can vary greatly from site to site, it is important to research each organization's programs, professional backgrounds of staff members, internship requirements, and other pertinent information well in advance of applying for an internship.

Although each internship location has its own admission criteria for prospective interns, many worksites typically place the greatest emphasis on a prospect's

- ability to perform basic health screenings (e.g., body fat, blood pressure, flexibility),
- grade point average of B or better in major field of study,
- evidence of a proven work ethic (e.g., volunteering, summer jobs),
- certification in first aid and CPR,
- good written and verbal communication skills, and
- evidence of a healthy lifestyle and image.

Some worksites have a specific application form for intern prospects to submit. A sample application may request

- information about your major and minor fields of study,
- your grade point average,
- the type of internship site desired (e.g., manufacturing industry, hospital, small business, managed care organization, community health organization, health club, rehabilitation center),
- certifications attained,
- dates of your proposed internship,
- number of weekly and total internship hours required by the university,
- major and minor courses completed,
- goals you would like to achieve in an internship,

## Internship Listing Organizations

For a listing of sample WHP-related internships, check out the following Web sites:

| | |
|---|---|
| www.hpcareer.net | www.internshipprograms.com |
| www.medicalfitness.org | www.wellnessconnection.com |
| www.internsearch.com | www.hfit.com/careers/internships.cfm |
| www.ltwell.com | www.cooperinst.org/intrn.asp |
| www.corporatefitnessworks.com | http://esmassn.org |
| www.exercisecareers.com | www.healthandwellnessjobs.com |

- your perceived strengths and weaknesses, and
- other information that you believe an internship supervisor and staff members should know about you.

For most students, an internship is the only real worksite experience they have before entering the job market. Thus, internship experiences should be carefully planned within a framework of clearly delineated policies and procedures. For example, I developed a Student WHP Manual that includes guidelines defining the relationship between student interns, university supervisors, and worksite supervisors. Here is a condensed version of these guidelines:

1. Most worksites require interns to have personal liability insurance coverage. This coverage is typically available through the university's personnel or human resources department at a very low cost.
2. The operating procedures of each internship are subject to both the worksite's discretion and the university's policies.
3. With rare exceptions, interns must pay their own living expenses.
4. Interns should experience the responsibilities of a full-time employee. Thus, a variety of activities are encouraged to foster an appreciation of the commitment required of a full-time job.
5. A university supervisor will usually visit the employer at least once to observe and discuss the intern's performance. Telephone conversations may replace on-site visits at distant locations.
6. The internship should last at least 10 weeks, with an average workload of 40 hours a week.
7. A successfully completed internship is equal to 12 semester hours of credit.

Sponsoring worksites and universities generally specify responsibilities for student interns. Some common work requirements for interns include the following:

1. Complete a basic orientation to the organization with a primary focus on
   - its organizational (administrative) hierarchy;
   - health promotion programs and services;

- WHP personnel training, certifications, and experience;
- problems, needs, and constraints for the existing health promotion program; and
- duties of an intern.

2. Participate in or observe a variety of ongoing activities such as staff conferences, workshops, seminars, and health fairs.
3. Complete the Planning and Evaluation Form before starting your major project; review it with the worksite supervisor on a regular basis.
4. If requested, toward the end of your internship, make a formal presentation of your internship experience to the worksite staff.

To fulfill written requirements for academic credit, the intern usually has the following responsibilities:

1. Keep a daily report of major activities and perceptions.
2. Prepare a weekly typed report (based on daily reports) that describes significant events and insights for each week. Give one copy to the worksite supervisor and send another to the university supervisor. The worksite supervisor and intern meet weekly to discuss each weekly report's contents and strategies for overall improvement.
3. Prepare a typed final report that includes both descriptive and analytical material. The first part should include descriptions of
   - the organizational structure of the company,
   - the purposes and goals of the company's health promotion program,
   - the program components and their functions,
   - the major sources of funding for the program, and
   - the project planning and evaluation.

The analytical overview of the internship should include insights on

- being a health promoter in a worksite setting,
- major benefits of the internship,

- suggestions for how the university might improve preinternship training experiences and future internship experiences, and
- how the worksite might improve the internship experience for future interns.

Upon completing your internship, submit two typed, bound copies of the final report—one to the worksite supervisor and one to the university supervisor. Their respective responsibilities are as follows:

*Common Responsibilities for Worksite Supervisors*

1. Provide the recommended orientation for the intern.
2. Assist in planning intern activities and supervising the intern during the internship.
3. Hold a weekly conference with the intern to discuss the intern's performance and specific recommendations for improvement.
4. Discuss the intern's performance with the university supervisor as needed.
5. Complete a mid-internship and final internship evaluation, and recommend a final grade to the university supervisor.

*Typical Responsibilities for University Supervisors*

1. Meet with the prospective intern on several occasions to determine career interests, skills, weaknesses; suggest specific preinternship preparatory experiences; explore worksite options; and coordinate the application process.
2. Clarify assignments and needs with the intern and worksite supervisor.
3. Make one or more visits to the worksite to review weekly reports and conduct mid-internship and final internship evaluations.
4. Obtain a letter-grade recommendation from the worksite supervisor, grade the intern's final report, and submit a final grade.

# JOB SEEKING

Because competition increases every year, you should position yourself for the future job market as early as possible. Register with the on-campus career placement office at least 6 months before you graduate to take advantage of various seminars on preparing application materials, interviewing tips, and job-seeking techniques. In addition, before graduating, be sure to do the following:

- During your internship, ask your internship supervisor how you can network with other WHP professionals on specific types of skills they're looking for in entry-level candidates and steps for enhancing your job-seeking efforts.
- Ask selective faculty members and your employer (if you are working) if they will serve as professional references for you.
- Check the Sunday edition of an area's major newspaper to review the classified section for employment opportunities relevant to your interests.
- Attend a state, regional, or national convention to network with prospective employers and use the on-site job placement center.
- Attend an on-campus job fair to network with prospective employers and participate in real or mock interviews.
- Check out various job listing sites on the Internet.

In the weeks and days before your interview, discover as much as you can about your potential future employer. Try to learn these specifics:

- Company size (number of employees and number of sites)
- Potential growth of the company
- Products, programs, and services the company provides
- Organizational structure of company headquarters and division offices or plants

## WHP Job Listing Web Sites

http://acsm.medcareers.com/seeker
www.healthpromotionjobs.com
www.hpcareer.net
www.phfr.com/jobFinder/seeker/search
www.wellnessjobs.com
www.exercisecareers.com
www.leisurejobs.com

- Management style (authoritative, participative, or a mixture)
- Union status (and relationship between union and management)
- Recent news about the company
- Company's health promotion philosophy
- Health promotion programs and facilities already in place
- Major health problems of an organization's workforce
- Organizational structure of health, fitness, and safety personnel; level of integration
- Potential growth of health promotion programs

You can find some of this information in the company's annual report, which may be available on the company's Web site or in a business directory at your local library (e.g., Standard & Poor's Directory).

Review the interview tips and recommendations that follow. Consider possible questions from the interviewer and rehearse you answers ahead of time. After practicing on your own, have a friend or classmate play the role of a prospective employer and ask you typical interview questions (along with a few surprise questions).

*Interview Like a Professional*

- Dress professionally, and arrive a few minutes early for the interview.
- Greet the interviewer with a handshake and pleasant smile.
- Maintain good posture and a calm disposition throughout the interview.
- In case your interviewer is not as organized as you are, bring along a clean copy of your resume for the interviewer to have on hand.
- Give the interviewer enough time to ask each question completely. Take time to think about the question before responding.
- Be honest about past and present employment activities, academic performance, courses taken, and perceived weaknesses or limitations.
- Avoid overusing technical terms; it is better to be perceived as down to earth than pretentious.
- Avoid using hand motions and other gestures to emphasize everything you say since they may be distracting to the interviewer.
- Send a letter of appreciation to the interviewer within 2 days after the interview.

## WHAT WOULD YOU DO?

You have just begun the final year of your academic program and meet with your advisor to discuss internship options. You would like to pursue an internship in a worksite that offers a comprehensive health and productivity management program, preferably in another city. Yet, in sharing your interest with the advisor, you feel his sense of such well-rounded internship experiences is quite limited because his primary focus is fitness center–based internships. To expand his knowledge of today's diversified internship marketplace while also taking personal responsibility for seeking a suitable internship, what would you do?

# Appendix A

## Personal Health Questionnaire

Please complete the following questionnaire and return it to _____. We will then contact you to schedule your first consultation. If you have any questions, please call _____.

*ALL INFORMATION IS CONFIDENTIAL*

Employee ID#: _____    Name: _____

Sex: ☐ M  ☐ F   Birthdate: _____   Dept./title: _____

Phone: Home ( ) _____    Work ( )_____

Emergency contact (name & phone #): _____ ( ) _____

### Activity Profile

Intensity and/or Exertion (please circle one)     Low          Moderate          High

   1. Level of physical activity at work.          1      2      3      4      5

   2. Level of physical activity at leisure.       1      2      3      4      5

   3. Do you currently exercise regularly?        ☐ No   ☐ Yes

   4. Number of times per week.                  1-2    3-4    5-6    Over 6

   5. How long do you exercise (minutes)?        <15    15-30   30-45   >45

   6. Briefly describe your exercise program: _____

_____

   If you answered No to question 3, when was the last time you exercised, and what type of activity did you do?

_____

_____

### Biomedical Profile

   1. Name(s) of your physician(s): _____

   2. Date of last complete medical exam: _____

   3. Do you know your resting blood pressure?   ☐ Yes   What is it? _____   ☐ No

   4. Do you know your resting heart rate?   ☐ Yes   What is it? _____   ☐ No

   5. Do you know your blood cholesterol level?   ☐ Yes   What is it? _____   ☐ No

   6. Do you know your ratio of total cholesterol to HDL cholesterol?
   ☐ Yes   What is it? _____   ☐ No

   7. Do you know your body fat percentage?   ☐ Yes   What is it? _____   ☐ No

*(continued)*

From *Worksite Health Promotion* by David H. Chenoweth, 2007, Champaign, IL: Human Kinetics.

Personal Health Questionnaire   *(continued)*

8. Do you have, or have you ever had, any of the following? Check all that apply.

| Condition | Past | Present | Condition | Past | Present |
|---|---|---|---|---|---|
| Angina | ☐ | ☐ | Rheumatic fever | ☐ | ☐ |
| Extra heartbeats | ☐ | ☐ | Dizziness/fainting | ☐ | ☐ |
| Arthritis | ☐ | ☐ | Scarlet fever | ☐ | ☐ |
| Heart attack | ☐ | ☐ | Emphysema | ☐ | ☐ |
| Asthma | ☐ | ☐ | Stroke | ☐ | ☐ |
| Heart murmur | ☐ | ☐ | Epilepsy | ☐ | ☐ |
| Back pain | ☐ | ☐ | Varicose veins | ☐ | ☐ |
| High blood pressure | ☐ | ☐ | Muscle weakness | ☐ | ☐ |
| Bronchitis | ☐ | ☐ | Muscle pain | ☐ | ☐ |
| Leg cramps | ☐ | ☐ | Bone injuries | ☐ | ☐ |
| Cancer | ☐ | ☐ | Bone pain | ☐ | ☐ |
| Pneumonia | ☐ | ☐ | Surgery* | ☐ | ☐ |
| Diabetes | ☐ | ☐ | Shortness of breath | ☐ | ☐ |

* Date of surgery: _____   Type of surgery:_____

9. Explanation/comments on any of the above: _____

_____

10. Other diseases/injuries/medical problems you have (past or present): _____

_____

11. Do you have any medical problem or injury that might make it difficult to exercise?  ☐ Yes  ☐ No

If yes, explain:_____

_____

## Family History

Indicate the number of blood relatives (mother, father, siblings) who have had:

| Condition | Number of relatives | Condition | Number of relatives |
|---|---|---|---|
| Alcoholism or drug addiction | _____ | Diabetes | _____ |
| Heart attack | _____ | High blood pressure | _____ |
| Heart attack before age 60 | _____ | Stroke | _____ |
| Obese (30% or more above ideal weight) | _____ | | |

## Health Inventory and Lifestyle

1. Height: _____   Weight: _____   Weight at age 21: _____

2. What do you consider to be a good weight for you? _____

3. Have you ever been on a diet prescribed by a doctor or registered dietitian?  ☐ No  ☐ Yes
   How many pounds did you lose? _____   In how many weeks? _____

4. Do you currently smoke tobacco products?  ☐ No    (Skip to #8)

    ☐ Yes    What type?  ☐ cigarettes; packs per day _____

                                ☐ cigars; number per day _____

                                ☐ pipe; pouches per day _____

5. How many years have you smoked? _____

6. What is the primary reason you smoke? _____

7. Have you ever tried quitting?  ☐ No   ☐ Yes   By what method _____

8. Do you drink alcoholic beverages?  ☐ No    (Skip to #9)

    ☐ Yes    What type:  ☐ beer; cans per day _____

                           ☐ wine; glasses per day _____

                           ☐ liquor; shots per day _____

9. What types of caffeinated beverages do you drink?

    ☐ caffeinated coffee; cups per day _____

    ☐ tea; glasses per day _____

    ☐ colas; cans per day _____

10. Place a check mark beside those foods you eat at least once a day.

    ☐ Whole milk        ☐ Hard cheese        ☐ Eggs        ☐ French fries

    ☐ Butter             ☐ Ice cream          ☐ Chocolate        ☐ Fast food

    ☐ Deep-fried foods    ☐ Cake/pie/doughnuts    ☐ Cold cuts     ☐ Chips

    ☐ Sausage/ham/bacon

11. How much stress do you have in an average day?

    ☐ More than the average person

    ☐ About the same as the average person

    ☐ Less than the average person

12. How do you manage stress? _____

## *Personal Interests*

Place a check mark beside the programs in which you would like to participate.

    ☐ Low-impact aerobics    ☐ Basketball      ☐ Smoking cessation

    ☐ Cycling                ☐ Bowling         ☐ Lifestyle management

    ☐ Low-back health       ☐ Softball         ☐ Parenting

    ☐ Nutrition             ☐ Volleyball      ☐ Caring for elders

    ☐ Weight control        ☐ Other (Please list)    ☐ Self-care

    ☐ Weightlifting         _____    ☐ Using health care benefits

    ☐ Walking             _____    ☐ Other (please list) _____

Thank you. Your feedback will help us plan programs and activities to help you achieve your personal health goals.

From *Worksite Health Promotion* by David H. Chenoweth, 2007, Champaign, IL: Human Kinetics.

# Appendix B

## Environmental Checksheet

### Nature of Work

1. Percentage of workers doing physical labor: _____%

2. Percentage sitting most of time: _____%

3. Percentage of workers

   standing: _____%    sitting: _____%    lifting: _____%

### Behaviors

1. Percentage of workers operating video display terminals (VDTs): _____%

   Are VDT stations equipped with

   ☐ filtered screens?    ☐ wrist/hand rests?    ☐ indirect lighting?

   Are they positioned appropriately for employees' height, reach, and posture? _____

   If not, what improvements are necessary? _____

2. Percentage of workers walking, standing, or sitting with poor posture: _____%

3. Percentage of workers doing a lot of lifting: _____%

   Percentage lifting over 10 pounds per lift: _____

4. Percentage of workers smoking

   on the job: _____%    in other areas where smoking may be permitted: _____%

5. Other significant behaviors (list):_____

### Environmental Health and Safety Hazards

1. Is the work environment noisy? _____

   If so, where? _____

2. Is the work environment    ☐ hot?    ☐ cold?

   If so, where? _____.

3. Is the lighting adequate? _____

   If not, where? _____.

4. Are fumes, vapors, or mists in the air? _____

   If so, describe: _____

5. Are employees exposed to substances that are toxic or caustic (burning)? _____

   If so, describe: _____

   Are employees properly protected? _____

*(continued)*

From *Worksite Health Promotion* by David H. Chenoweth, 2007, Champaign, IL: Human Kinetics.

6. Are employees around flying objects? _____

    If so, where? _____

    Are employees properly protected? _____

7. Are employees likely to injure themselves due to excessive lifting or improper lifting? _____

    If so, where? _____.

8. Are any areas slick (oily, wet)? _____

    If so, where? _____.

9. Do areas exist where employees may fall? _____

    If so, where? _____.

10. Do any areas exist where employees may be caught in, on, or between machinery? _____

    If so, where? _____.

## Safety Promotion and Injury Prevention

1. Are warning devices posted at high-risk areas? _____

    If not, where needed? _____

2. Are visible posters displayed to motivate safety practices? _____

    If not, where needed? _____

3. Are safety records posted? _____

    If not, what is a central location for all employees to see? _____.

4. Do workers in high-risk areas wear proper clothing, safety gloves, hard hats, goggles, protective shoes? _____

    If not, where are they needed? _____

## Summary

1. Nature of work for most employees is ☐ physical or ☐ mental.

2. Most significant behaviors displayed among workers include:

    A. _____

    B. _____

    C. _____

3. Degree of risk associated with health and safety hazards:

    A. High _____*

    B. Fair _____*

    C. Low _____

    *Reasons: _____

    _____

Signature (Investigator): _____ Date: _____

# Bibliography

## Chapter 1

Association for Worksite Health Promotion, Mercer, W.M., Inc., and U.S. Department of Health and Human Services. (1999). *1999 National worksite health promotion survey: Report of survey findings.* Northbrook, IL.

Burton, W., Chen, C., Conti, D., Schultz, A., and Edington, D. (2003). Measuring the relationship between employees' health risk factors and corporate pharmaceutical expenditures. *Journal of Occupational and Environmental Medicine,* 45(8), 793-802.

Burton, W., Chen, C., Schultz, A., and Edington, D. (1999). The cost of body mass index levels in an employed population. *Statistical Bulletin, Metropolitan Life Insurance Company,* 80(3), 8-14.

Cowan, C., Catlin, A., Smith, C., and Sensenig, A. (2004). National health expenditures, 2002. *Health Care Financing Review,* 25(4), 143-146.

Durbeck, D., Heinzelmann, F., Schacter, J., et al. (1972). The National Aeronautics and Space Administration—U.S. Public Health Service Health evaluation and enhancement program. *American Journal of Cardiology,* 30, 784-790.

Edington, D., and Yen, L. (1992). Is it possible to simultaneously reduce risk factors and excess health care costs? *American Journal of Health Promotion,* 6, 403-409.

*Employee Benefit News.* (2005). Health care costs remain execs' No. 1 concern. February 1, page 1.

Employee Services Management Association. (2004). Hot trends. News release, August. [www.esmassn.org/trends/].

Goetzel, R., Anderson, D., Whitmer, R., Ozminkowski, R., Dunn, R., and Wasserman, J. (1998). The relationship between modifiable health risks and health care expenditures. *Journal of Occupational and Environmental Medicine,* 40(10), 843-854.

*HERO Forum for Optimal Employee Health,* e-newsletter. (2005). Health Enhancement Research Organization. May 17.

Kaiser Family Foundation (2002). *Trends and indicators in the changing health care marketplace, 2002 Chartbook.* Derived from Centers for Medicaid and Medicare Services, Office of the Actuary.

Kirsten, W. (2005a). International Health Promotion Resources (2005). *WELCOA's Absolute Advantage,* 4 (4), 26-29.

Kirsten, W. (2005b) Second annual European health and productivity congress. *Health & Productivity Management,* 4 (3), 33-35.

The MEDSTAT Group MarketScan Database. (1997). Diabetes: A cost driver in employee health plans. *Business & Health Special Report,* December, 4-8.

Milliman & Roberson, Inc. (1995). *Health risks and their impact on medical costs.* A study by Milliman and Robertson, Inc., in conjunction with the Chrysler Corporation and the International Union of Auto Workers, Brookfield, WI.

*National Health Expenditure (NHE) historical estimates and projections.* (2004). National Health Statistics Group, Office of the Actuary, Centers for Medicare & Medicaid Services (CMS). November 1.

Okada, K., and Muto, T. (2005) Total health promotion in Japan: A successful model at Osaka Gas Company. *WELCOA's Absolute Advantage,* 4(4), 26-28.

Pronk, N., Goodman, M., O'Connor, P., and Martinson, B. (1990). Relationship between modifiable health risks and short-term health care charges. *Journal of the American Medical Association,* 282, 2235-2239.

Rundle, R. (2002). Obesity tops smoking for medical costs. Rand Corporation. *The Wall Street Journal,* March 12, B7.

Stead, B. (1994). Worksite health programs: A significant cost-cutting approach. *Business Horizons,* November-December, 37(6), 73-76.

Texas Instruments. *Texins: A look back.* [www.texins.org/history.htm].

Thompson, S. (2003). Worksite wellness programs on the USA-Mexico border. *California Journal of Health Promotion,* 1(4), 102-108.

The World Bank. (2005). Population Changes in the World. World Development Indicators. [http://web.wordbank.org].

Zeidner, R. (2004). Fitness on the job. *The Washington Post,* August 17, HE01.

## Chapter 2

Cox, C. (2003). *ACSM's worksite health promotion manual: A guide to building and sustaining healthy worksites.* Champaign, IL: Human Kinetics.

Gilmore, G., and Campbell, M. (2005). *Needs and capacity assessment strategies for health education and health promotion,* 3rd ed. Sudbury, MA: Jones and Bartlett.

Pelletier, B. (2003). Intelligent innovations. *WELCOA's Absolute Advantage,* 2(8), 46-51.

Society of Prospective Medicine. (1976). New concepts in health: A new horizon. Proceedings of the twelfth annual meeting, Society of Prospective Medicine, October 1, San Diego, CA.

## Chapter 3

Agoglia, J. (2005). The AED agenda. *Club Industry's Fitness Business Pro*, February, 32-35.

Carrier, K. (2004). Seeing things through different eyes. *WELCOA's Absolute Advantage*, 3(7), 17-19.

Centers for Disease Control and Prevention. (2004). Diagnoses of HIV/AIDS – 32 States, 2000-2003. *Morbidity and Mortality Weekly Report*, 53(47), 1106-1108.

Chenoweth, D. (2002). *Evaluating worksite health promotion*. Champaign, IL: Human Kinetics.

Curry, S., Ludman, E., and McClure, J. (2003). Self-administered treatment for smoking cessation. *Journal of Clinical Psychology*, 59(3), 305-319.

Eisenberg, M. (2000). Is it time for over-the-counter defibrillators? *Journal of the American Medical Association*, 284, 1435-1438.

Gmelich, T. (2000). Defibrillators and health and fitness clubs: Member benefit or liability risk? *ACSM's Health & Fitness Journal*, 4(5), 27-28.

Glanz, K., Lewis, F., and Rimer, B. (1997). *Health behavior and health education: Theory, research, and practice*, 2nd ed. San Francisco: Jossey-Bass.

Glasgow, R., Hollis, J., Ary, D., and Boles, S. (1993). Results of a year-long incentives-based worksite smoking-cessation program. *Addictive Behaviors*, 18(4), 83-104.

Hennrikus, D., Jeffery, R., Lando, H., et al. (2002). The SUCCESS Project: The effect of program format and incentives on participation and cessation in worksite smoking cessation programs. *American Journal of Public Health*, 92(2), 274-279.

Lenert, L., Munoz, R., Stoddard, J., et al. (2003). Design and pilot evaluation of an Internet smoking cessation program. *Journal of the American Informatics Association*, 10(1), 16-20.

Robison, J. (2004). Toward a New Science. *WELCOA's Absolute Advantage*, 3(7), 3-5.

Seaward, B. (2004). The path to spiritual wellness. *WELCOA's Absolute Advantage*, 3(7), 12-15.

Smedslund, G., Fisher, K., Boles, S., and Lichtenstein, E. (2004). The effectiveness of workplace smoking cessation programmes: A meta-analysis of recent studies. *Tobacco Control*, 13(2), 197-204.

*The Wall Street Journal*. (2005). Insurers consider covering smoking programs. April 26, D1 and D6.

Tully, S. (1995). America's healthiest companies. *Fortune*, June 12, 98-106.

Wik, L., Kramer-Johansen, J., Myklebust, H., et al. (2005). Quality of cardiopulmonary resuscitation during out-of-hospital cardiac arrest. *Journal of the American Medical Association*, 293, 299-304.

Wilson, M., Holman, P., and Hammok, A. (1996). A comprehensive review of the effects of worksite health promotion on health-related outcomes. *American Journal of Health Promotion*, 10, 429-435.

## Chapter 4

American Cancer Society. (2003). *Cancer Facts and Figures 2003*, page 25. [1-800-ACS-2345].

Brown, J., and Kellerman, A. (2000). The shocking truth about automated external defibrillators. *Journal of the American Medical Association*, 284, 1438-1441.

Cardinal, B. (2004). Employee maintenance: Worksite health promotion programs are a sound business investment. *American Fitness*, 22(12), 40-43.

Cash, G. (1996). Financial wellness: Will it be your next health promotion program? [www.healthy.net/library/articles/cash/center/worksite.htm].

Cherry, D., and Woodwall, D. (2002). *National ambulatory medical care survey: 2000 summary*. National Center for Health Statistics. Advance Data from Vital and Health Statistics, Number 28, June 5, p. 1.

Fichtenburg, C., and Glantz, S. (2002). Effect of smoke-free workplaces on smoking behaviour: Systematic review. *British Medical Journal*, 325, 1188-1191.

Johnson, D. (1997) Renovation. *Fitness Management*, 4, 30-32.

Kadowaki, T., Watanabe, M., Okayama, A., Hishida, K., and Ueshima, H. (2000). Effectiveness of smoking cessation intervention in all of the smokers at a worksite in Japan. *Industrial Health*, 38, 396-403.

Kadowaki, T., Kanda, H., et al. (2006) Are comprehensive environmental changes as effective as health education for smoking cessation? *Tobacco Control*, 15(1), 26-29.

Kellett, K., Kellett, D., and Nordholm, L. (1991). Effects of an exercise program on sick leave due to back pain. *Physical Therapy*, 71, 283-293.

Maher, C. (2000). A systematic review of workplace interventions to prevent low back pain. *Journal of Physiotherapy*, 46, 259-269.

Robison, J., and Carrier, K. (2004). *The spirit and science of holistic health*. [www.authorhouse.com].

*WELCOA's Absolute Advantage*. (2005). Work & stress in America: Reversing the vicious cycle. 3(8), 3-5.

## Chapter 5

Burke, R., and Robson, R. (1995). In and outsourcing: How to assess vendors. *AWHP's Worksite Health*, 1, 14-16.

Doniek, C., and Sattler, T. (1998). Planning & preparing a budget. *Fitness Management*, July, 28.

Sattler, T., and Doniek, C. (1995). How to choose trouble-shooting consultants. *Fitness Management*, 11, 40-41.

## Chapter 6

Burke, T. (1988). The economic impact of alcohol abuse and alcoholism. *Public Health Reports*, 103(6), p. 567.

Cady, L., Thomas, P., and Karwasky, R. (1985). Program for increasing health and physical fitness of firefighters. *Journal of Occupational Medicine*, 27, 110-114.

Hilyer, J., Brown, K., Sirles, A., and Peoples, L. (1990). A flexibility intervention to reduce the incidence and severity of joint injuries among municipal firefighters. *Journal of Occupational Medicine*, 32, 631-638.

Kaman, R. (Ed.). (1995). *Worksite health promotion economics*. Champaign, IL: Human Kinetics.

Pronk, N. (2004). Addressing multiple risk factors at the worksite. *ACSM's Health & Fitness Journal,* 9(5), 28-31.

Proschaska, J., Norcross, J., and DiClemente, C. (1994). *Changing for good*. New York: William Morrow and Company.

Sirles, A., Brown, K., and Hilyer, J. (1991). Effects of a back school education and exercise in back injured municipal workers. *Journal of the American Association of Occupational Health Nursing*, 39, 7-12.

Thompson, D. (1990). Effect of exercise breaks on musculoskeletal strain among data-entry operators: A case study. In *Promoting Health and Productivity in the Computerized Office* by Steven Saulter et al., pp. 118-127. New York: Taylor and Francis Publishers.

## Chapter 7

Atkinson, W. (2001). Is wellness incentive money well spent? *Business & Health,* May, 23-27.

Chenoweth, D. (2002). *Evaluating worksite health promotion*. Champaign, IL: Human Kinetics.

Chenoweth, D. (2001). Decision points around evaluation. *AWHP's Worksite Health*, Summer, 8-14.

Healthcare Information and Management Systems Society. (2002). E-Health: Navigating the Internet for health information (White Paper). Chicago, IL. [www.hipaadvisory.com/action/ehealth/himss.pdf].

Edington, D. (2004). How health risk appraisals can take your program to the next level (interview with Wellness Councils of America, Part I). [www.welcoa.org].

HIPAA. (2001). Overview of the proposed regulations. *Federal Register*, 66(5), January 8.

Landro, L. (2005). Web grows as health-research tool. *The Wall Street Journal*, May 18, D7.

Pronk, N. (2004). Addressing multiple risk factors at the worksite. *ACSM's Health & Fitness Journal,* 9(5), 28-31.

Proschaska, J., Norcross, J., and DiClemente, C. (1994). *Changing for good*. New York: William Morrow and Company.

Reeves, M., and Rafferty, A. (2005). Healthy lifestyle characteristics among adults in the United States, 2000. *Archives of Internal Medicine*, 165, 854-857.

Sullivan, N. (2002). 5 factors for success: byte size advice for e-health management. *WELCOA's Absolute Advantage*, 2(1), 14-17.

What Is the ADA: Definition of disability obtained from www.adata.org/whatsada-definition.aspx, May 30, 2005.

Wegleitner, T. (2002). The fundamentals: A model for worksite health promotion. *WELCOA'S Absolute Advantage*, 2(7), 14-17.

Williams, V. (2004). Team coaching for company success. *WELCOA's Absolute Advantage*. 3(9), 21-23.

## Chapter 8

Chenoweth, D. (2002). *Evaluating worksite health promotion*. Champaign, IL: Human Kinetics.

Chenoweth, D., Martin, N., Pankowski, J., and Raymond, L. (2005). A benefit-cost analysis of a worksite nurse practitioner program: First impressions. *Journal of Occupational & Environmental Medicine*, 47(11), 1111-1116.

Chenoweth, D., and Garrett, J. (2006). Cost-effectiveness analysis of a worksite clinic: Is it worth the cost? *Journal of the American Association of Occupational Health Nursing*, 54(2), 84-89.

Kirsten, W. (2005). A healthy world. *WELCOA's Absolute Advantage Magazine*, 4(4), 20-25.

Suchman, E. (1967). *Evaluative research*. New York: Russell Sage Foundation.

## Chapter 9

Anderson, D. (2003). Right on target: A WELCOA expert interview. [www.davidhunnicutt.com/pdf/Anderson_interview.pdf].

Association for Worksite Health Promotion, Mercer, W.M., Inc., and U.S. Department of Health and Human Services. (1999). 1999 National worksite health promotion survey: Report of survey findings. Northbrook, IL: William M. Mercer.

Chenoweth, D. (1995). Health promotion in small business. In *Critical Issues in Worksite Health Promotion*, Mark Wilson and David DeJoy (Eds.), Chapter 12. Needham Heights, MA: Allyn & Bacon.

COSEwell Wellness Program. [www.cose.org].

*Healthy Workforce 2010: An essential health promotion sourcebook for employers, large and small*, Partnership for Prevention, Fall 2001. [www.prevent.org. products/benefits].

McMahan, S., Wells, M., Stokols, Phillips, K., and Clitheroe, H. (2001). Assessing health promotion programming in small businesses. *American Journal of Health Studies*, 17(3), (Summer), 120-128.

Medrea, J. (1995). How Champion merged health and family services into its business plan. *AWHP's Worksite Health*, (Winter), 32-35.

U.S. Department of Health and Human Services. (1993). 1992 national survey of workplace health promotion activities: Summary. *American Journal of Health Promotion*, 7, 452-464.

Wilson, M., DeJoy, D., Jorgensen, C., and Crump, C. (1999). Health promotion programs in small worksites: Results of a national survey. *American Journal of Health Promotion*, 13, 358-365.

## Chapter 10

AWHP Professional Standards Task Force. (1995). How do you measure up? Guidelines for the worksite health promotion director. *AWHP's Worksite Health*, 2(3), 18-23.

Jones, J., and Ver Voort, G. (1995). What employers want: UWSP-AWHP survey results. Presentation at the American Alliance for Health, Physical Education, Recreation and Dance National Convention, April 17.

Karch, R., and Rose, M. (2004). Measuring up. *WELCOA's Absolute Advantage*, 3(3), 46-49.

Rojas-Guyler, L., Cottrell, R., and Wagner, D. (2006). The second national survey of U.S. internship standards in health education professional preparation: 15 years later. Poster session, American Alliance for Health, Physical Education, Recreation and Dance National Convention, April 26.

Stevenson, M., Bachtel, J., and Moeller, M. (2004). Retooling without reschooling. *WELCOA's Absolute Advantage*, 3(3), 42-45.

Snelling, A. (2004). The journey...from good to great. *WELCOA's Absolute Advantage*, 3(3), 37-41.

# Index

Note: The italicized *f* and *t* following page numbers refer to figures and tables, respectively. The italicized *ff* and *tt* following page numbers refer to multiple figures and tables, respectively.

# About the Author

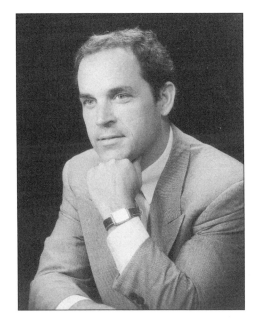

As a professor of health education and director of worksite health promotion studies at East Carolina University, the author has taught, advised, and supervised undergraduate and graduate students since 1979.

He has written several books, including *Health Care Cost Management: Strategies for Employers* and *Evaluating Worksite Health Promotion*. A fellow of the Association for Worksite Health Promotion (AWHP), Dr. Chenoweth served as the education/university chair for AWHP Region II, from which he received the President's Award in 1995. He serves on the medical advisory board of the Wellness Councils of America (WELCOA) and chaired the Business and Industry committee of the North Carolina Governor's Council on Physical Fitness and Health for 14 years. He has made many presentations on health promotion and health care cost management issues to various organizations throughout the United States and conducted seminars on worksite health promotion to the Jamaican Ministry and the European Union.

As president of Chenoweth & Associates, Inc. he provides strategic consulting, data analysis, and econometric evaluation services to public and private organizations. He served as the chief econometric analyst in the development of a physical inactivity cost calculator with Active Living Leadership and has conducted risk factor cost analyses for eight states.

Dr. Chenoweth received his PhD from The Ohio State University and his BS and MA degrees from Ball State University. He and his wife, Katie, and son, Zach, live in New Bern, North Carolina. In his leisure time, he enjoys golfing, biking, and landscaping.

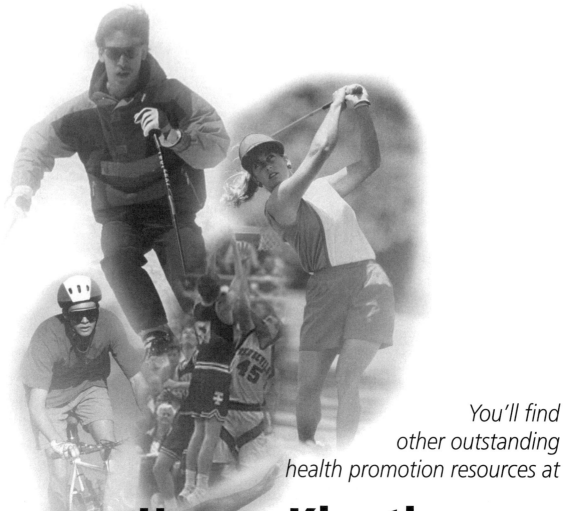

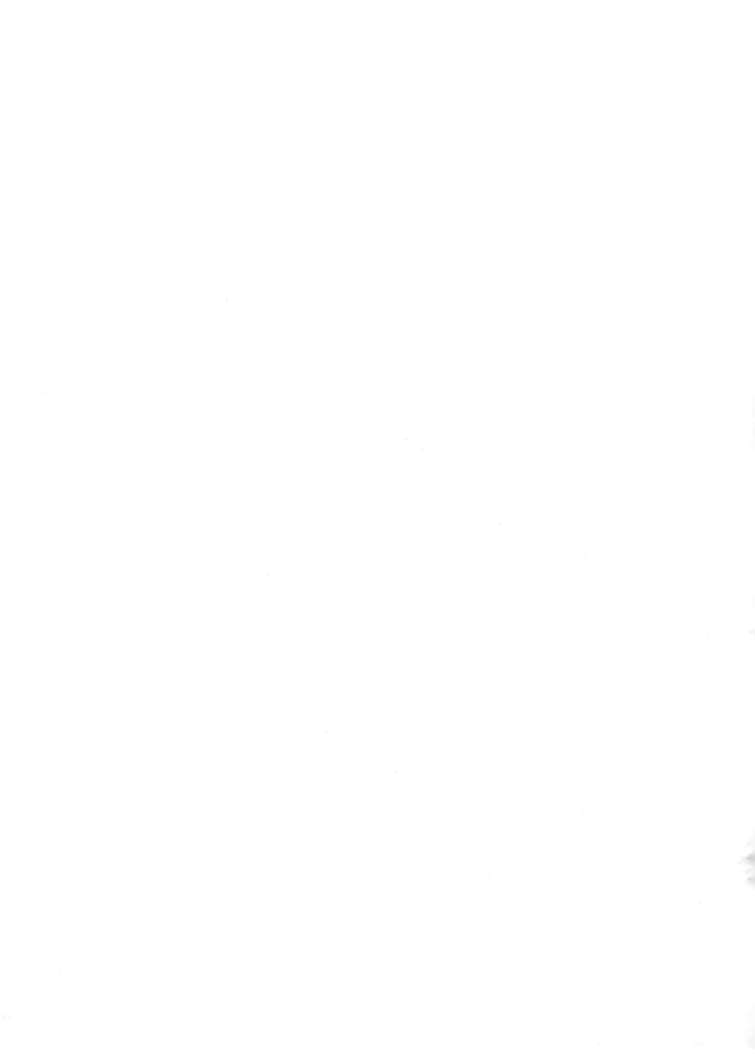